CONCEPTUAL MODELS

OF NURSING:

ANALYSIS AND APPLICATION

Joyce J. Fitzpatrick, Ph.D., F.A.A.N.
Professor and Dean
Frances Payne Bolton School of Nursing
Case Western Reserve University
Cleveland, Ohio

Ann L. Whall, Ph.D., F.A.A.N.
Associate Professor
College of Nursing
Wayne State University
Detroit, Michigan

Robert J. Brady Co. • *Bowie, Maryland 20715*
A Prentice-Hall Publishing and Communications Company

Executive Editor: Richard A. Weimer
Production Editor: Janis K. Oppelt
Art Director: Don Sellers AMI
Assistant Art Director: Bernard Vervin
Cover Designer: Don Sellers AMI
Text Designer: Paula K. Aldrich
Typeface: Trump
Typesetting & Pasteup: Prestige Editorial and Graphics Services, Inc.
                        Washington, D.C.
Printed by: Fairfield Graphics
            Fairfield, Pennsylvania

Conceptual Models of Nursing: Analysis and Application

Library of Congress Cataloging in Publication Data
Main entry under title:

Conceptual models of nursing.

   Bibliography: p.
   Includes index.
   1. Nursing—Philosophy. I. Fitzpatrick,
Joyce J., 1944–   II. Whall, Ann L., 1935–
[DNLM: 1. Nursing process.   2. Models, Theoretical.
WY 100 C7445]
RT84.5.C664   1983   610.73'01   82-17913
ISBN 0-89303-233-6

Prentice-Hall International, Inc., London
Prentice-Hall Canada, Inc., Scarborough, Ontario
Prentice-Hall of Australia, Pty., Ltd., Sydney
Prentice-Hall of India Private Limited, New Delhi
Prentice-Hall of Japan, Inc., Tokyo
Prentice-Hall of Southeast Asia Pte. Ltd., Singapore
Whitehall Books, Limited, Petone, New Zealand
Editora Prentice-Hall Do Brasil LTDA., Rio de Janeiro

Printed in the United States of America

83 84 85 86 87 88 89 90 91 92 93   10 9 8 7 6 5 4 3 2

CONTENTS

FOREWORD

Organization and development of nursing knowledge is required for effective transmission in selected, ordered learning experiences and for effective selection and utilization of knowledge in professional practice. A clear conceptualization of nursing is one essential component of any rational, cognitive structure for the organization and development of nursing knowledge.

Products of today's theorists or model builders are only the most recent, and perhaps more formalized, statements to explicate the nature of nursing in a long heritage. Persistent themes of a holistic view of humans, of valuing individuality, of safeguarding dignity and worth in spite of sickness, debility, helplessness, or poverty, and of nursing as a distinctive humanitarian helping of a particular type are apparent in the heritage. To understand, evaluate, utilize or amend, and develop today's models a nurse must know the heritage and the evolutionary context. Nurses must be able to make comparative analyses.

Statements on the nature of nursing have ranged from definitions to "theories." So called theories are sometimes expressions of beliefs and values, of visions, and of global noble goals for shaping the future. Some are models or first approximations of a system of concepts with recognizable empirical referents to explicate what nursing is thought to be. This mixture of philosophical or belief stances with structures intended for the processes and products of science contributes to the confusion evident in nursing literature from the multiple meanings of the terms *theory, nursing,* and *nursing theory.* This confusion is furthered by the intermingling of nursing as practice and that of the knowledge basic to that practice.

These editors and authors have provided a text useful for sorting out some of the confusion. They also provide an opportunity for organized study of the significant conceptualizations of nursing that have shaped or are shaping American nursing. The book provides a presentation of each conceptualization of nursing along with insights to influences and values for individual theorists. The scheme for analysis applied throughout the book provides a basis for contemplating adequacy in meanings, scope, consistency, and cohesion of the particular models. One can also consider the models for their contributions, potentials, and implications for nursing practice, nursing education, and nursing research.

The compilation provides a useful base from which to grow. It is an essential base for understanding nursing conceptually. It provides substance for recognizing similarities, variations, gaps, issues, and inadequacies in explicit ideas about nursing. Only with awareness of these can nurses meet responsibilities for improvements in utilization, transmission, and development of knowledge of nursing.

Rosemary Ellis, Ph.D., R.N.
Professor of Nursing
Frances Payne Bolton School of Nursing
Case Western Reserve University
Cleveland, Ohio

PREFACE

This book grew out of our involvement in the discovery of nursing knowledge. It represents several years of teaching and learning, of uncovering the historical roots upon which nursing, as science and art, is based, and of tracing relationships between and among theoretical developments proposed by nursing's scholars. Our goal is to share our perspective on the development of nursing knowledge by analysis of the nursing models and theories that have been presented over the years in the literature.

In our opinion two features of this book are unique: the use of consistent guidelines for analysis of each of the models and the Comparative Charts of Nursing Models which crystallize the essential components of each model. Dr. Barbara Pieper, contributor of Chapter 7, is responsible for providing the idea for the chart which was enthusiastically adopted by other chapter contributors. It is our expectation that both of these special components will add to the usefulness of the book. Budding scientists are encouraged to explore the relationships in the models that exist and, ultimately, to create new understandings of nursing.

All of the contributors to the book have been students of mine from whom I have learned much about these nursing models. Each of the contributors has added depth and breadth to the analyses, evaluations, and applications included here. The learning atmosphere was rich at the Wayne State University College of Nursing, where, in the doctoral level theory courses, we developed and molded our ideas. We are all indebted to our colleagues in this endeavor, faculty and students whose contributions are only indirectly reflected in this book, those who questioned us and, therefore, encouraged us by their questioning, and those who supported us enthusiastically to pursue this endeavor. This book was seven years in its development. It spans the period of time from 1975-1982 when I developed and taught the nursing theory courses, as I developed my visions of nursing, and as I refined my theoretical understandings that are presented here in Chapter 17. These understandings are presented for the first time in the form of a theoretical model for nursing, and they are offered as beginning tenets toward a broad understanding of the scientific focus of nursing. It is hoped that they will generate critique and, ultimately, lead to more extensive and more rigorous tests of the tentative hypotheses.

It is our expectation that this book will be most useful to students involved in beginning theory analysis endeavors. At the same time, graduate students and faculty may find it particularly useful because of its comprehensive nature. It is hoped that as new ideas emerge during our scientific quest in nursing we may all continue to share our theoretical insights.

Joyce J. Fitzpatrick

CONTRIBUTORS

Claire M. Andrews, Ph.D., C.N.M., R.N.
Associate Professor, Frances Payne Bolton School of Nursing
Case Western Reserve University
Cleveland, Ohio

Suzanne H. Brouse, M.S., R.N.
Doctoral Candidate, College of Nursing
Wayne State University
Detroit, Michigan

Veronica Engle, Ph.D., R.N.
Assistant Professor, School of Nursing
University of Wisconsin-Madison
Madison, Wisconsin

Joyce J. Fitzpatrick, Ph.D., F.A.A.N.
Professor & Dean, Frances Payne Bolton School of Nursing
Case Western Reserve University
Cleveland, Ohio

Paula J. Gonot, M.S., R.N.
Doctoral Student, College of Nursing
Wayne State University
Detroit, Michigan

Ruth L. Johnston, Ph.D., R.N.
Associate Professor, College of Nursing
Rutgers-The State University
Newark, New Jersey

Shirley Cloutier Laffrey, Ph.D., R.N.
Assistant Professor, School of Nursing
University of California—San Francisco
San Francisco, California

Carol J. Loveland-Cherry, Ph.D., R.N.
Nurse Researcher
Ann Arbor, Michigan

Barbara A. Pieper, Ph.D., R.N.
Assistant Professor, College of Nursing
Wayne State University
Detroit, Michigan

Jana L. Pressler, M.A., R.N.
Doctoral Student, Frances Payne Bolton School of Nursing
Case Western Reserve University
Cleveland, Ohio

Stephanie I. Muth Quillin, M.S., R.N.
Doctoral Candidate, College of Nursing
Wayne State University
Detroit, Michigan

Edith D. Raleigh, Ph.D., R.N.
Nurse Researcher
Harper-Grace Hospitals
Detroit, Michigan

Pamela G. Reed, Ph.D., R.N.
Assistant Professor, College of Nursing
University of Arizona
Tuscon, Arizona

Judith Aumente Runk, M.Ed., R.N.
Assistant Director for Continuing Education
William Beaumont Hospital
Royal Oak, Michigan

Mary E. Tiedeman, M.N., R.N.
Doctoral Student, College of Nursing
Wayne State University
Detroit, Michigan

Ann L. Whall, Ph.D., F.A.A.N.
Associate Professor, College of Nursing
Wayne State University
Detroit, Michigan

Sharon A. Wilkerson, Ph.D., R.N.
Director of Nursing Research
St. Joseph's Mercy Hospital in Pontiac
Pontiac, Michigan

S. Joy Winkler, Ph.D., R.N.
Associate Professor, School of Nursing
McGill University
Montreal, Quebec

Tamara L. Zurakowski, M.A., R.N.
Doctoral Student, Frances Payne Bolton School of Nursing
Case Western Reserve University
Cleveland, Ohio

1

OVERVIEW OF NURSING MODELS AND NURSING THEORIES

Joyce J. Fitzpatrick & Ann L. Whall

The professional practice of nursing is based on scientific knowledge. This scientific focus within nursing demands attention to theory development and research, and the relationship between them. In their scientific quest, nurses have developed a base of knowledge which has substantially shaped the nursing perspective and which has guided educational programs, research, and professional practice. The scientific heritage of contemporary nursing is rich in resources. While there is indeed diversity among the many scientific statements of the nature of nursing, there clearly emerges a perspective of nursing that characterizes the field of inquiry.

Nursing science is focused on the elaboration of relationships between person and environment in relation to health. Nursing interventions may or may not be formally explicated within the scientific domain. The existence and elaboration of practice theory has in fact remained an unresolved issue within nursing.

THEORY PERSPECTIVES WITHIN NURSING SCIENCE

Theory development as a process has been highlighted as a significant area of study for scientists within nursing. Concomitant with this focus on theory development has been an attention

to the usefulness of the knowledge generated in guiding professional practice. It can be concluded that the most critical need for
advancement of the profession of nursing is the development,
elaboration, and substantiation of the scientific base.

The structure of science, in part, theory development and research, exists to achieve the goals of understanding and prediction (Dubin, 1978). While these goals are complementary, the
specific theory development and research processes which lead
to their achievement may seem conflicting at specific junctures
or points of analysis. Understanding as a goal of science frequently leads to broad generalizations that demonstrate general
relationships among the phenomena of concern. Prediction as a
goal of science more concertedly directs one to specificity in
statements of relationships.

Theory development in nursing is concerned with both understanding and prediction. The range of specificity of theoretical
formulations within nursing science varies greatly. To some extent this range has broadened as nursing has sought to answer the
complex questions that confront an emerging profession. Beginning with the nineteenth century scientific and professional
leadership of Florence Nightingale, nursing, as a scientific discipline, reflects a rhythm in the process of theory development. A
pattern of peaks or conceptual breakthroughs can be observed as
one scans the forest. While it is of great importance toward overall scientific development to maintain the perspective of the forest, it is equally imperative that the discipline evaluate the nature
of the trees. The similarities among oaks, pines, and maples
assists in understanding the more general phenomena. An overall
perspective of nursing has been identified (Donaldson and Crowley, 1978; Fawcett, 1978; Fitzpatrick, Whall, Johnston and Floyd,
1982). The objective remains to further describe, analyze, and
evaluate the specifics.

In summary, nursing is on the brink of an exciting new era.
The two decades preceding the eighties found nursing theorists
debating such now dated questions as: should there be one conceptual framework for nursing; what types of nursing research
should be encouraged; and, is nursing a basic or an applied science? This self-reflection has influenced the development of both
new and old conceptual frameworks and has fostered research
based upon the frameworks, research guided by the frameworks,
and educational programs and practice protocols based upon the
frameworks. From the work of Nightingale to that of the more
recent theorists, e.g. King, Orem, Rogers, and Roy, these concep-

tual models or conceptual frameworks* have become familiar to nurses from all levels of educational preparation. The excitement of the eighties and nineties concerns the involvement by all of nursing, not just nurse theorists, with the nursing conceptual models. As more nurses become familiar with these models or use them to guide education, research, and practice, the need to systematically assess each model becomes more vital. Although the models are not in and of themselves considered theories, they lead to the development of theories relevant to nursing.

Commonalities and differences among the nursing conceptual models should be assessed to highlight consistencies and to generate scientific debate. The way in which this scrutiny takes place needs to be at least twofold. That is, a scrutiny of the conceptual models should use terms which are understandable to large numbers of nurses who use the frameworks and at the same time, the scrutiny should use terms and procedures useful to nurse theorists. The analysis guidelines presented in this text seek to highlight relevant points of analysis and a few points of evaluation. Certainly there are numerous other points which may be considered, and which are included in other guidelines, but the guidelines used in this text sought to achieve a measure of simplicity to enhance understanding of the comparisons.

The analysis guidelines used throughout this text were developed by Fitzpatrick and used by beginning doctoral students for analysis of nursing models.** The guidelines compare the nursing conceptual models—which vary in levels of abstractness as well as completeness—by addressing each model in a separate chapter. The models are presented in chronological order, generally arranged by decade, from the oldest to the newest.

Models included were judged to be those most influential in the shaping of nursing knowledge. A historical approach is taken as the nursing perspective of Nightingale is first analyzed. This is followed by analysis of the models presented in the 1950s and 1960s including those of Peplau, Orlando, Wiedenbach, Henderson, Levine, Johnson, and Orem. The models presented in the 1970s, including Roy, Zderad and Patterson, and Neuman, King,

---

*Conceptual models and conceptual frameworks are terms used interchangeably in this work.
**Acknowledgment is given to Margaret A. Newman, Ph.D., F.A.A.N., whose instruction greatly influenced the development of these guidelines.

Rogers, and Newman are then analyzed. As an introduction to
the 1980s, the model of Parse is analyzed and the beginning
developments of Fitzpatrick's model and its analysis are presented. The final chapter is focused on theory development for
the future of nursing science.

There are several points which need to be made before the
guidelines are presented. There are debates concerning the nursing conceptual models which are relevant to this discussion. One
current debate concerns what the nursing conceptual models are
to be named: are these theories, theoretical frameworks, conceptual frameworks, or conceptual models? The editors use the term
"nursing models," for the most part and have based the rationale
for this decision upon the following discussion.

The literature on theory development in nursing continues
to address the differences between theories and conceptual
frameworks. It is generally accepted that conceptual frameworks
or models provide a way of viewing nursing. Conceptual models
are thus general statements of the phenomena with which a discipline is concerned. The linkages between concepts of a model
are not always evident (Hardy, 1978). A theory, on the other hand,
is more specific and consequently more closely related to reality.
The conceptual linkages are more evident. The differences between conceptual models and theories thus have in part to do
with both level of abstraction as well as degree of explication.
These differences are now well accepted.

There is also debate about how to analyze and evaluate a
nursing model. Although there are several ways to analyze and
evaluate models, by way of beginning it is useful to review the discussion of Kaplan's (1964) and Jacox's (1974) approach. Kaplan
has identified that there is a theoretical-empirical continuum. At
one pole, the more concrete terms are represented or concepts
which deal with directly observable phenomena. Terms which
deal with infections might, for example, be placed at this end of
the continuum. At the opposite pole can be placed terms or concepts which deal with phenomena which cannot directly or
indirectly be observed. Such concepts as health and environment
are what Kaplan would call constructs, and "theories" using constructs might also be placed at the most abstract pole of the continuum. Jacox defines constructs as terms which are made up of
several types of concepts, and are what Dubin would call summative units which stand for an entire complex of a thing (Dubin,

1978). As such, the entire complex of environment cannot be directly or indirectly observed. Dubin states that "theories" (his term) which use, primarily, summative units are not directly testable.

The nursing models in large part are composed of summative units. These terms and thus the models need to be further elaborated and specified toward the development of testable theories. A theory, according to Ellis (1968), is a coherent set of interrelated concepts, hypotheses, and principles which forms a general frame of reference. The nursing models are not generally, however, to this level of specificity from which law-like principles may be derived and tested. But as descriptions derived from empirical data and relevant knowledge, the models can and do guide practice, serve as conceptual frameworks for nursing research, and also serve as a proper object of nursing research in which the concepts are analyzed and further defined and the relationships explicated.

Because the nursing models in general are not yet to the level of specificity of theory as defined by Ellis, theory analysis systems are not for the most part appropriate to use. It is noted, however, that portions of certain models, such as that of Peplau (1952), appear to approach a theoretical level. A special approach, therefore, needs to be used to evaluate and analyze nursing models by drawing upon several analysis systems. These considerations were used in developing the guidelines discussed below.

GUIDELINES FOR ANALYZING NURSING MODELS

The guidelines presented here are primarily analysis guidelines for conceptual models. As such they ask the question appropriate to conceptual models. For example, rather than addressing the testability of a theory, the usefulness of the model is addressed. Each chapter uses the same guidelines presented in Table 1.1, which serves as the organizing scheme for each chapter; this should assist in comparison between models. Thus, each chapter included in this book addresses model analysis in the same basic manner. The chapters include attention to the basic concepts of person, environment, health, nursing, and analysis of internal and external model components.

Table 1.1

Guidelines for Analyzing Nursing Models

I. Introduction

II. Basic considerations included in the model
    A. Definition of person, nursing, health, environment
    B. Description of nursing activity
    C. Understanding of person
    D. Understanding of health
    E. Interrelationships among concepts of person, environment, health, and nursing
    F. Description of the basic concepts included in this model
    G. Relationships of basic concepts of person, environment, health, and nursing

III. Internal analysis and evaluation
    A. Underlying assumptions
    B. Central components of the model
    C. Definitions of these components
    D. Relative importance of components
    E. Relationships among components
    F. Analysis of consistency
    G. Analysis of adequacy

IV. External analysis of the model
    A. Relationship to nursing research
    B. Relationship to nursing education
    C. Relationship to professional nursing practice

V. Summary

INTRODUCTION

Each chapter presents a statement regarding the background of the model. Briefly, the way in which the theorist was influenced in her thinking or came to develop her model is described. The amount of background material which is available varies so that some variation between chapters necessarily occurs in the type and amount of background material presented.

ANALYSIS OF BASIC CONSIDERATIONS

The time between Nightingale's nineteenth century model statement, the mid-twentieth century statement of Peplau and Henderson, and the contemporary nursing models was characterized by many societal changes. Surprisingly, however, both Nightingale and the twentieth century theorists address the same basic concepts either explicitly or implicitly of person, environment, health, and nursing. In this section, the author analyzes, or examines, the elements of the model. Because the four concepts of person, environment, health, and nursing are generally considered basic to, and either implicitly or explicitly stated in all nursing models, these concepts receive preliminary examination. These questions are addressed: What are the definitions of these concepts, and more than this, what is the understanding of these concepts basic to the model? What are the relationships among these concepts? Finally, because this text emphasizes the analysis of the model for scientists, educators, and practitioners, the questions relating to explication of nursing activities receive emphasis. Besides addressing the definition and the understanding of the concept of nursing, the authors discuss the description of the nursing activities.

INTERNAL ANALYSIS AND EVALUATION OF THE MODEL

In this section the analysis is taken a step further, and portions of the model are analyzed, examined, and evaluated. This overall assessment is focused on internal adequacy. These questions are addressed: What are the implicit and explicit assumptions of this model? How do the implicit and explicit assumptions relate to each other? Then, because each nursing model contains concepts (components) specific to the model, the specific model concepts are analyzed. These questions are addressed: What are the central components of the model? What is the relative importance of the components? What type of concepts are used according to Dubin (1978)? What are the definitions of these components and what are the relationships among components (if these are evident)? Propositional statements of specific relationships between concepts that are included in these models are

identified. Finally, the evaluation questions are addressed. Specifically, these questions are asked: What is the internal consistency of the model? That is, are the concepts clearly defined
and/or defined in more than one way? Are the concepts used in
consistent ways throughout the model? Are the assumptions consistent with the concepts and the relationships between concepts? Other evaluation questions are those identified by Hardy
(1974) and Ellis (1968). Although the questions identified by
Hardy and Ellis are those more specific to theories and not models, the questions are posed because some of the nursing models
approach, in part or in general, a theoretical level. The questions
borrowed from Hardy are: What is the meaning and logical adequacy of the model? Specifically, the logic and implications of the
assumptions and the meaning of the concepts are addressed.
Then, operational adequacy is addressed: Are there operational
definitions for the concepts, are these adequate, and may
hypotheses be drawn from the model? It is important to point out
that because constructs (i.e., summative units) cannot be
operationally defined without considerable work and inference,
the majority of models will not meet this criteria. Since most
models are not for the purpose of prediction and are at a high level
of abstraction, the other criteria which Hardy addresses—
pragmatic adequacy, generality, and predictability—are not
addressed. The following section on external analysis reflects
consideration of additional criteria. Ellis' (1964) questions, which
are relevant to model analysis, are then addressed to complete the
internal evaluation of the model. These questions are: What is
the scope of the model? (Scope, according to Ellis, refers to the
number of smaller concepts which are covered in the model; the
broader the scope the greater the potential significance for nursing.) What is the complexity of the model? (Simple postulations
which are readily apparent are not particularly valuable to nursing in Ellis' view.) What is the usefulness of the model? That is,
can the model be used to guide clinical practice? Finally, does the
model generate new information? In Ellis' view, even relationships which are difficult to test can contribute significantly to
understanding if they stimulate new ways of viewing old
problems.

EXTERNAL ANALYSIS OF THE MODEL

In this last section, the authors consider external criteria in
assessing the model. Three basic questions are addressed: What is

the relationship of the model to nursing research? What is the relationship of the model to nursing education? What is the relationship to professional practice? These questions are focused not only on what currently exists, but also on the potential that is inherent in the model for research, education, and professional practice. The first question addresses the way in which the model might guide research and/or specific examples of ways in which the model might guide and has guided educational programs are discussed. Finally, the way in which the model might guide professional practice is discussed and in some chapters, a practice example is addressed.

SUMMARY

In this section the important points of both the analysis and evaluation are highlighted. This serves as a concise statement of the chapter's contents.

It is hoped that this model analysis guideline will stimulate comparisons by scientists and practitioners which will lead to further development, refinement, and use of these models. Comparisons can be made and commonalities and differences identified through the study of these chapters. A major inclusion in this book *is the insert,* which presents a summary of each of the theorists' condensed statements regarding person, health, environment, and nursing. This summary is designed not only to present in crystallized form the essential contributions of each model to the science of nursing, but also to spur comparative analysis among current nursing scholars.

In summary, the book, while focused on analysis of the various nursing models, barely uncovers the tip of the iceberg in the scholarly arena of nursing. The challenge for scientific development is clear. At best, this overall analysis of the nursing perspective will lead to scholarly discussion and debate which will clearly advance the science of nursing.

REFERENCES

Donaldson S, Crowley D: The discipline of nursing. Nursing Outlook, Vol 2, pp 113-120, 1978
Dubin R: Theory Building. The Free Press, New York, 1978
Ellis R: Characteristics of significant theories. Nursing Research, Vol 17, No 3, pp 217-222, 1968

Fawcett J: The what of theory development. *In* Theory development: What, why, and how. National League for Nursing, New York, 1978

Fitzpatrick JJ, Whall AL, Johnston RL, Floyd JA: Nursing Models and Their Psychiatric Mental Health Applications. Robert J. Brady, Bowie, Maryland, 1982

Hardy M: Theories: Components, development, evaluation. Nursing Research, Vol 23, No 2, pp 100-107, 1974

Hardy M: Evaluating nursing theory. *In* Theory Development: What, Why, and How. National League for Nursing, New York, 1978

Jacox A: Theory construction in nursing. Nursing Research, Vol 23, No 1, pp 4-12, 1974

Kaplan A: The Conduct of Inquiry. Harper and Row, New York, 1963

Newman, M: Theory Development in Nursing. F.A. Davis Co., Philadelphia, Pennsylvania, 1979

Peplau H: Interpersonal Relations in Nursing. G.P. Putnam's Sons, New York, 1952

2

NIGHTINGALE: A VISIONARY MODEL FOR NURSING

Pamela G. Reed & *Tamara L. Zurakowski*

INTRODUCTION

Florence Nightingale was the forerunner of nursing theory development in that her "laws of nursing," also referred to as laws of health or nature, provided the earliest perspective for defining nursing (Nightingale, 1859/1969). Nightingale's conceptual model is a compilation of "laws" which describe the relationships between the concepts of nursing, person, environment, and health, and address activities designed to alter a person's environment for restoration or promotion of health. Analysis and application of the "laws of nursing," Nightingale believed, would promote well-being and relieve the suffering of humanity (Cook, 1942; Murphy, 1978; and Schlotfeldt, 1977).

It is suggested that nursing began its scientific base when Nightingale identified these "laws of nursing" (Barritt, 1973). However, it must be noted that Nightingale's view of nursing encompassed a somewhat different and broader perspective than what is typically regarded as professional nursing today. A nurse was, to Nightingale, any woman who had the "charge of the personal health of somebody," whether sick or well (p 3, 1859/1969). She held a religious view of nursing as a "calling," or God's work. The nurse was to acquire and apply knowledge about God's laws

11

of health and, thus, move humankind closer to perfection. Nursing activities served as an art form through which spiritual development might occur (Cook, 1942; Grace, 1978). Her *Notes on Nursing* were written to offer "hints for thought" and encourage all women to learn about the laws of health through observation and experience.

A brief review of Nightingale's life reveals four major factors that operated to influence her model of nursing: religion, science, war, and feminism. She was born to an English aristocratic family on May 12, 1820, during the Victorian era. It was a time when it was not normative for women to display intelligence, assertiveness, or any interests beyond domestic or social events. Nightingale frequently attempted escape from what she considered the futility of this female, aristocratic role through daydreaming, visits with the sick and poor, her own physical ills, and, at times, contemplation of suicide (Cook, 1942; Huxley, 1975). Nightingale was well-educated, an experienced traveler, spoke several languages, and pursued the meaning of life, truth, and the will of God through religious and philosophical studies. She frequently interacted with leading scientists and educators of her day.

Implications by Bullough (1979) and Ehrenreich and English (1973) that Nightingale turned to nursing out of the frustrated maternal needs of a spinster are not consistent with Nightingale's or others' depiction of nursing. Nightingale was one who vehemently objected to the female Victorian role of indolence and marriage, and viewed the development of nursing as a "respectable livelihood and constructive social utilization of women" (Palmer, 1977). Nursing activities were not undertaken out of submission to the physician or merely a motherly devotion to the patient as implied by Enrenreich and English (1973). The activities were to be based not only on compassion, but also observation and experience, statistical data, knowledge of sanitation and nutrition, and administrative skills (Agnew, 1958; Andrews, 1929; Barritt, 1973).

BASIC CONSIDERATIONS
INCLUDED IN THE MODEL

Notes on Nursing represented Florence Nightingale's first effort at putting her philosophy and description of nursing in one written source. Prior to its publication, she had limited her nursing literature to pieces of personal correspondence. Nightingale's ideas also appeared in the form of personal letters and pamphlets which were distributed to influential governmental officials.

Definition and Description of Nursing

Nightingale describes two different types of nursing, sick nursing or "nursing proper," and health nursing (p 127, 1859/ 1969; 1893/1949). All women were to practice health nursing, which required some practical teaching, and the goal of which was prevention of disease. It was for health nurses that *Notes on Nursing* was originally written, although the text was later used in the Nightingale school. The bases for health nursing were the laws of life and health. Both sick nursing and health nursing were to "put the patient in the best condition for nature to act upon him" (Nightingale, p 133, 1859/1969).

Nursing proper was both an art and a science, and required an organized, scientific, and formal education (Nightingale, 1893/ 1949) to care for those suffering from disease. The scientific dimension grew from Nightingale's own grasp of statistics, sanitation, logistics, administration, and public health, as well as the laws of health and symptoms of disease. Nightingale (1893/1949) was explicit in defining nursing as distinct from medicine, citing nursing's concern with the patient who was ill, rather than the illness, as the basic difference. Although nurses were to carry out physician orders, they were to do so only with an independent sense of responsibility for their actions.

Description of Nursing Activity

The focus of nursing activity for both health nurses and trained nurses was the proper use of "fresh air, light, warmth, cleanliness, quiet, and the proper selection and administration of diet" (Nightingale, p 8, 1859/1969), while monitoring the patient's expenditure of energy. Activity was to be directed toward the patient's environment as well as the patient.

Trained nurses required specialized knowledge in addition to the laws of health for their wider scope of practice (Nightingale, 1893/1949). Prescribed content in the Nightingale school included, among other things, observing the sick, bandaging, making occupied beds, applying leeches, using surgical appliances, managing the convalescing, and preparing gruel, arrowroot, egg flip, puddings, and drinks for the sick (Nightingale, 1882b/1954; 1893/1949).

The goals of nursing activity were broad; they included maintenance of health, prevention of infection and injury, recovery from illness, health teaching, and environmental control (Nightingale, 1859/1969; 1893/1949). Moreover, one did not need to be ill to benefit from nursing knowledge; nor did one have to be wealthy. The laws of nursing had the potential to better everyone's lot in life.

Definition and Description of Person

Nightingale envisioned the person as comprised of physical, intellectual, emotional, social, and spiritual components. She viewed all persons as equal, transcending biological differences, socioeconomic class, creed, and disease. Although Nightingale's laws of health focus primarily on the physical dimensions of the patient, she presented ideas on the psychology of suffering. Some examples are that the sick have a more vivid imagination than the well, the sick benefit from hearing about pleasant events, and the sick are like children in that there is no proportion in events to them (Nightingale, pp 95-104, 1859/1969).

The centeredness of the patient in Nightingale's (1859/1969) model is evidenced in her emphasis upon the natural course of events which work in the patient to effect cure. This is facilitated by environmental factors, activities of the nurse, and the medicine and surgery of the physician (p 133). Nightingale viewed the person as having both the ability and responsibility to alter rather than conform to the existing situation. Such efforts, Nightingale believed, would relieve spiritual and physical suffering and improve conditions for both the individual and the community (Cook, 1942; Palmer, 1977).

Definition and Description of Environment

The environment, in Nightingale's model, refers to those physical elements external to the patient which affect the healing process and health such as noise, air, temperature, and other meaningful stimuli. Her laws of nature operationally define ways by which the environment could affect the patient's health. An example of these laws is: Keep the air within the patient's room as pure as the outside air through the proper use of fuel and ventilation (Nightingale, pp 12-20, 1859/1969). Other laws refer to using lids on chamber crockery, rinsing utensils, cleaning carpets and curtains, and restricting inappropriate consolation and conversation.

Nightingale's regard for the patient's enviornment as a major concept in her model emerged, in part, out of her early Crimean war experiences with the sickness and death that occurred as a result of unsanitary environmental conditions of the wounded and sick soldiers at Scutari. However, Nightingale attributed these conditions to "dirt, damp, draughts, drains, drink, and diet" and not to germs or microorganisms. In fact, she was deeply concerned that attention to "mystic rites" such as antiseptics and disinfectants would sway people from the real problem (Nightingale, 1893/1949). The significance of environment is reflected in Torres' (1980) reference to Nightingale's model as an "Environmental Theory of Nursing" (p 28).

Nightingale consulted and wrote extensively on the organization, construction, and management of hospitals (Bishop, 1960). It may be stated that her greatest insight into the importance of the environment in the preservation of health is evidenced in her concern for the "health of houses" and her claim that one could better predict health problems if one checked "houses, conditions, ways of life" rather than the physical body (Nightingale, p 123, 1859/1969). Although Nightingale disregarded Lister's theoretical postulations about disease and germs, her recommendations for hospitals were based largely on meticulously tabulated statistics on the outcomes of hospitalized patients.

Definition and Description of Health

Health is an additive process, the result of environmental, physical, and psychological factors. In particular, the environmental factors of "dirt, drink, diet, damp, draughts, and drains" affect health (Nightingale, p 362, 1893/1949). Health is considered not only as the opposite of disease, but includes being "able to use well every power we have to use" (Nightingale, p 334-335 1882b/1954). Disease, according to Nightingale, is a reparative process that is the body's attempt to correct some problem. She also believed that being diseased provided one an opportunity to gain spiritual perspective (Nightingale's letter of April, 1873, in Cook, 1942).

INTERNAL ANALYSIS

Underlying Assumptions

Nightingale's approach to model building aids in understanding assumptions basic to her model. Both "experiential" and "spectator" knowledge were essential to Nightingale, but, as Maslow (1966) supports, the former had priority in her search for truth. This is to say, abstract ideas about nursing, health, or environment were grounded upon experience and were to be reformulated if they were found to be inconsistent with the empirical world.

Nightingale regarded observations that were based on one's senses as the only reliable means for obtaining and verifying knowledge (Palmer, 1977; Schlotfeldt, 1977). She practiced and taught nursing based on the realities as she saw them, and admonished nurses to "let experience not theory" be their guide (Levine, 1963; Nightingale, pp 76, 122, 1859/1969). She assumed that things not verified by the senses were superstition, and therefore rejected the principles of bacteriology, antisepsis, and germs (Huxley, 1975). Moreover, Nightingale proclaimed that nothing, not even the miracle of the Resurrection, should be exempt from criticism and accepted without sufficient evidence (Barritt, p 9, 1973).

Nightingale's approach to model development involved the organization of experiential knowledge into empirical generalizations primarily through inductive reasoning. Nightingale's process of theory development resembles the participant-observer approach described by Ellis (1969) and Quint (1967), whereby the "laws of nursing" were generated from practice and experience. Theory that was not grounded in practical experience was, to Nightingale, mere "inspiration" (Cook, 1942).

Central Components:
Definitions and Relationships

There are four central components in Nightingale's model: 1) Nursing—a calling, the goal of which is to discover and use nature's laws governing health in the service of humanity; 2) Person—one with physical, intellectual, and metaphysical attributes and potentialities; 3) Health—to be well and able to use every power one has; and 4) Environment—those elements external to and which affect the health of the sick and healthy person. These concepts are identified as "summative" units (Dubin, 1978) in that they are global and nonspecific in their representation of reality. For example, the concept "environment" represents everything from the patient's food and flowers to the nurse's verbal and nonverbal interactions with the patient. "Nursing" encompasses a wide range of activities related to putting the patient in the best possible condition for nature to cure. Thus, there is a great deal of variability in the potential meanings of these major components. Nightingale's laws of nursing, however, serve to elucidate in concrete terms some of the meanings of these abstract components.

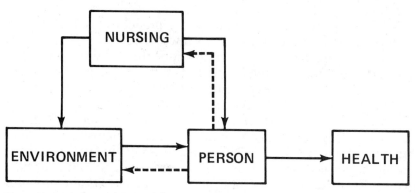

Figure 2.1. Nightingale's Model.

The relationships among the components are explicit for the most part. The diagram depicts the *person* as having the key role in his or her health. *Nursing* contributes to the person's ability to regain or maintain health either directly or indirectly through management of the person's *environment. Health* is a function of the interaction between nursing, person, and the environment. Nightingale identifies unidirectional relationships between nursing and person, and between nursing and environment, in that nursing activities are directed toward altering the environment and affecting the patient. Neither the environment nor the person are clearly presented as influencing the nurse.

Less explicit are the relationships between person and environment, and between person and nurse. Although Nightingale outlines several environmental factors which affect the person, she does not delineate the individual's influence upon the environment, or upon the nurse. The patient is regarded almost as a passive receptacle who is affected by nurse and environment.

However, she does credit the person with the ability and responsibility to better his/her environment. In addition, Nightingale implies an interrelation between person and nursing in her description of the nurse as modifying the activities according to the patient's abilities to help himself or herself and to change the environment.

Analysis of Consistency

Nightingale's model is judged in general to have internal consistency in that the relationships among the major concepts are consistent and flow logically from the meaning attributed to each concept (Hardy, 1974).

The organization of Nightingale's model follows what Reynolds (1971) describes as the "set of laws" theory; that is, her "laws of nursing" are empirical generalizations that outline knowledge about the existence of relationships between concepts, but do not propose substantive explanation about how the phenomena occur. Set-of-laws (Reynolds, 1971) indicates only that the concepts have the potential for measurement, and does not imply causality. It is the most rudimentary form of theory, and usually requires further research. The causal form of theory, in contrast to the set-of-laws form, provides for some understanding of how concepts relate to each other in a variety of contexts and provides information needed to make some predictions about the consequences of a given relationship. The causal process allows for hypothetical concepts whereas the set-of-laws is dependent upon observable occurrences. Thus, the set-of-laws approach to model building is consistent with Nightingale's assumptions about the experiential basis of knowledge. For example, Nightingale's model does not explain *how* such environmental factors as sunlight, fresh air, or quietness function to promote health; rather, it states only that these factors are related.

Analysis of Adequacy

A criterion for adequacy of meaning is that the concepts are presented in a manner similar to that of other scientists (Hardy, 1974). The validity of the meanings attributed to the concepts of the model is borne out by Nightingale's and others' explications of her success in improving the health of patients. These positive outcomes also give evidence for the empirical adequacy of Nightingale's model; that is, the relationships among the concepts as proposed by her were supported in her actual practice with sick individuals. For example, improvement of environmental conditions at Scutari dramatically reduced the mortality rate.

The logical adequacy of Nightingale's model cannot be sufficiently determined because the magnitude of the relationships is not specified; the linkages between concepts cannot be formalized in a way described by Hardy (1974). For example, sunlight and cleanliness are proposed to promote health but no linkage is made between the two environmental factors such that one can be identified as more effective than the other, or so that two can be determined to have greater impact on health than one.

The laws of health provide concrete examples of the major concepts of nursing and environment in particular and contribute to the operational and empirical adequacy of the model. Many of the laws or empirical generalizations presented in Nightingale's *Notes on Nursing* are at a testable level of abstraction. For example, the following empirical generalizations can be tested: clean air, sunlight, and quiet in a person's environment promote health; chattering hopes of visitors fatigue a patient; unnecessary contact with a patient's bed is a painful annoyance; and form, color, and variety, e.g., flowers, improve physical and mental well-being (Nightingale, 1859/1969). Without the empirical generalizations, however, the concepts themselves are too abstract to be tested or applied to practice; to "use well every power" one has is not a measurable description of the concept, health.

The numerous laws within Nightingale's model expand the scope of the model. The model is comprised of a number of related observations and facts. However, it lacks complexity in that the postulations are readily apparent (Ellis, 1968). The laws describe observable events but do not propose hypothetical explanations as to why certain relationships exist and they do little to stimulate new insights, although at the time they were revolutionary (Woodham-Smith, 1951). Because the model lacks complexity, its usefulness in the clinical setting is limited to particular contexts which resemble Nightingale's patients' situations, e.g., physically sick persons who could substantially benefit from provisions of sunlight and fresh air.

In spite of these deficits, Nightingale's model meets the criteria proposed by Hardy (1978) for grand level theory or theory which consists of broad terms and is at a high level of abstraction. The conceptual model provides a perspective for the nursing discipline by employing meanings and theoretical terms that are close to common usage and by offering empirical data to illustrate the basic concepts.

EXTERNAL THEORY ANALYSIS

Nightingale's bias toward use of experiential data in discovering the basic "laws of nursing" contributed to the identification of the four major components which have since provided the perspective for the development of nursing models capable of guiding nursing practice, education, and research. The adequacy of the Nightingale model, however, limits the direct application of her concepts in practice and research.

Relationship to Nursing Research

Nightingale's delineation of research as relevant and essential to nursing has continuing implications for nurse researchers (Barritt, 1973). She acknowledged that, while the "laws of nursing" were as yet unknown, nurses had to be "truthseekers" and continue discovering the "great secrets of nursing" (Montiero, 1974). Nightingale's work estblished a definition and focus of inquiry, which is the starting point for any research.

Palmer (1977) identifies recording, communicating, order and codification ability, conceptualization, inference, analysis, and synthesis as the essential research strengths that Nightingale possessed. She engaged in historical, explanatory, descriptive, comparative, and field research. Nightingale identified the model presented in *Notes on Nursing* as the result of data she had collected during the Crimean War and in the fourteen years following it (1859/1969). Torres (1980) suggests that the more recent work on stress, need, and adaptation are closely related to Nightingale's conceptualization.

Although Nightingale's conceptualization is exemplary, her approach to building knowledge can be criticized by today's standards of theory development. It seems likely that she viewed "truth seeking" and practice as concurrent activities, an idea considered inappropriate by Walker (1971), who states that the relationship between practice and theory building must clearly differentiate between those goals and activities concerned with the development of theoretical knowledge and those concerned with the deliberate use of knowledge, i.e., those activities of the theorist and the practitioner, respectively. The failure to distinguish between these two types of activities can limit the knowledge which "truth seeking" could ultimately offer clinical practice.

Relationship to Nursing Education

Nightingale's influence on nursing education can still be observed in many ways, and has been undiscovered in others. She insisted upon scientifically-based content, to be taught by faculty members with varying backgrounds and expertise. Nursing education was to follow a general education, and students were encouraged to attend the theater and concerts (Barritt, 1973). Nightingale included all of these ideas in the school of nursing at St. Thomas' Hospital, which opened in 1860. Assignments still in use today, e.g., case studies and clinical logs ("ward diaries"), had their beginning at St. Thomas'.

Nightingale also advocated that schools of nursing have administrative and economic structures that were independent of those of the hospital. Underlying this was a belief that students were there to learn, not to provide service. The hospital was to function as a place for students to practice their newly-learned nursing skills. Only recently had this come to pass in the United States.

Nightingale was very clear about her position on both entry into practice and continuing education for nurses. Formal education was regarded simply as that which taught nurses how to go on learning for themselves and provided only basics (Nightingale, p 332, 1882a/1954). The formal educational experience was to reflect the different careers in nursing. That is, hospital nurses—those who would care for the ill in institutions—should receive one year of schooling. District nurses who provided primary health care, midwives, and those who sought leadership or administration roles in hospitals required three years of education. Her opposition to licensure resulted in part from her concern that qualities important in nurses could not be assessed on a single examination and that it was dangerous to give people unlimited license to practice. While her stand on licensure is not applicable to today's professional standards, Nightingale's concerns about adequate evaluation methods and the need for continuing education are highly relevant in nursing education today.

Relationship to Professional Practice

Nightingale's model can be viewed as a practice theory, defined by Dickoff, James, and Wiedenbach (1968) as one which seeks to shape reality and contains the necessary components of goal-content, prescriptions, and survey lists. Nursing was a part of a larger goal of improved health and education for the entire British populace (Kelly, 1976). Toward this end, Nightingale encouraged nurses to be intellectual and creative in the delivery of nursing care. These ideas are still pertinent today.

The realm of nursing practice includes the spiritual, physical, emotional, mental, and social needs of the patient (Nightingale, 1859/1969; 1867; 1893/1949). No pathology need be present for one to benefit from nursing care. Nightingale was explicit in defining nursing knowledge as distinct from medical knowledge, and nurses as independent from physicians (Nightingale, pp 9-10, 131-133, 1859/1969). Later statements seem to contradict this, as Nightingale wrote that nursing was the "skilled servant of medicine, surgery, and hygiene" (Nightingale, p 335, 1882b/1954) and compared nurses to "the building staff" and physicians to the "architect" (Cook, p 270, 1942). These remarks were likely aimed at appeasing the physicians who complained that Nightingale's nurses were over-educated. Her comment was perhaps more a reflection of her socio-political skills rather than a definitive statement on nursing.

Nightingale's most important message to practitioners lies in her understanding of how nursing is related to the whole of society, including social and political contexts. For example, effective nursing practice required a liberal education, intellectual and reasoning powers, adequate pay, and support systems. Auxiliary personnel, properly taught, were considered a resource for nurses since they could free a nurse to carry out her duties. More importantly, the specialized knowledge of nurses dictated that they be supervised and supported only by other nurses. Nightingale (1893/1949) was clear in conveying that progress in nursing was the ongoing responsibility of nurses.

SUMMARY

Over one hundred years after Nightingale published her work, nurses continue to argue over essential issues—professional autonomy, licensure and certification, continuing education, and entry into practice. Florence Nightingale developed an early but significant model from which such issues can be addressed. She identified the wholistic nature of the individual and a variety of ways in which the environment was important.

Health was defined as encompassing more than a lack of disease. Nightingale's model may be considered a beginning theory of nursing, as described by Ellis (1968), in that it is directed toward helping individuals in their health needs and seeks to guide nursing practice. The scope of the model is broad enough to remain relevant to nursing. It lacks the complexity, however, to generate specific testable hypotheses. Additionally, the links between concepts are at times undefined. It is not useful to dwell on these criticisms of Nightingale's model, however, since it is inappropriate to apply current criteria for evaluation of a theory to the earliest conceptualization of professional nursing. Although bound in part by the context of her era, Nightingale's dedication to discovering "laws of health" for the purpose of benefitting the sick and healthy, and her awareness of the significance of the social and physical environment for patients and nursing as a whole, initiated a trend toward the development of what is recognized today as the discipline of nursing.

REFERENCES

Agnew LRC: Florence Nightingale—statistician. American Journal of Nursing, Vol 58, No 5, pp 664-665, 1958

Andrews MRS: A Lost Commander: Florence Nightingale. Doubleday, Doran, Co., New York, 1929

Barritt ER: Florence Nightingale's Values and Modern Nursing Education. Nursing Forum, Vol 12, No 1, pp 7-47, 1973

Bishop WJ: Florence Nightingale's message for today. Nursing Outlook, Vol 8, No 5, pp 246-249, 1960

Bullough B: The expanding role of the registered nurse. In JR Folta and ES Deck (eds): A Sociological Framework for Patient Care, 2nd ed, John Wiley & Sons, Inc., New York, pp 142-152, 1979

Cook E: The Life of Florence Nightingale (Vols I and II). The MacMillan Co., New York, 1942

Dickoff J, James P, Weidenbach E: Theory in a practice discipline. Part I: Practice-oriented theory. Nursing Research, Vol 17, No 5, pp 413-435, 1968

Dubin R: Theory Building (Rev Ed). The MacMillan Co., New York, 1978

Ehrenreich B, English D: Witches, Midwives, and Nurses—A History of Women Healers, 2nd ed. The Feminist Press, Old Westbury, New York, 1973

Ellis R: Characteristics of significant theories. Nursing Research, Vol 17, No 3, pp 217-222, 1968

Ellis R: The practitioner as theorist. American Journal of Nursing, Vol 69, No 7, pp 1434-1438, 1969

Grace HK: The development of doctoral education in nursing: A historical perspective. In NL Chaska (ed): The nursing profession, McGraw-Hill Book Co., New York, pp 112-123, 1978

Hardy ME: Theories: components, development, evaluation. Nursing Research, Vol 23, No 2, pp 100-107, 1974

Hardy ME: Evaluating nursing theory. In Theory Development: What, Why, How?, National League for Nursing, New York, pp 75-86, 1978

Huxley E: Florence Nightingale. G.P. Putnam's Sons, New York, 1975

Kelly LY: Our Nursing heritage: Have we renounced it? Image, Vol 8, No 3, pp 43-48, 1976

Levine ME: Florence Nightingale: The legend that lives. Nursing Forum, Vol 2, No 4, pp 24-35, 1963

Maslow AH: The Psychology of Science. Henry Regnery Co., Chicago, Illinois, 1966

Montiero LA (ed): Letters of Florence Nightingale. Nursing Archive, Boston, Massachusetts, 1974

Murphy J: Toward a philosophy of nursing. In NL Chaska (ed): The nursing profession, McGraw-Hill Book Co., pp 3-9, New York, 1978

Nightingale F: Notes on Nursing: What It Is and What It Is Not. Dover Publications, Inc., New York, 1969, (Originally published, 1859)

Nightingale F: Suggestions for the improvement of the nursing service of hospitals and on the method of training nurses for the sick poor. Reprinted from Blue book: Report on cubic space in metropolitan workhouses, 1867

Nightingale F: Training of nurses. In LR Seymer (ed): Selected writings of Florence Nightingale, The MacMillan Co., New York, 1954, (Reprinted from A dictionary of medicine, R Quain (ed), Originally published, 1882a)

Nightingale F: Nursing the sick. In LR Seymer (ed): Selected writings of Florence Nightingale, The MacMillan Co., New York, 1954, (Reprinted from A dictionary of medicine, R Quain (ed), Originally published, 1882b)

Nightingale F: Sick nursing and health nursing. In IA Hampton (ed): Nursing of the sick, 1893, McGraw-Hill Book Co., New York, 1949, (Originally published, 1893)

Palmer IS: Florence Nightingale: Reformer, reactionary, researcher. Nursing Research, Vol 26, No 2, pp 84-89, 1977

Quint JC: The case for theories generated from empirical data. Nursing Research, Vol 16, No 2, pp 109-114, 1967

Reynolds PD: A Primer in Theory Construction. Bobbs-Merrill Co., Inc. Indianapolis, Indiana, 1971

Schlotfeldt RM: Nursing research: Reflection of values. Nursing Research, Vol 26, No 1, pp 4-9, 1977

Torres G: Florence Nightingale. *In* Nursing theories: The base for professional nursing practice. Prentice-Hall, Inc., Englewood Cliffs, New Jersey, 1980

Walker LO: Toward a clearer understanding of the concept of nursing theory. Nursing Research, Vol 20, No 5, pp 428-434, 1971

Woodham-Smith C: Florence Nightingale. Constable and Co. Ltd., London, England, 1951

3

PEPLAU'S NURSING MODEL: THE INTERPERSONAL PROCESS

Pamela G. Reed & Ruth L. Johnston

INTRODUCTION

Prior to discussing the Peplau conceptual model of nursing, it seems appropriate first to view the historical background and social situation in which Hildegarde Peplau first published a more formalized definition of nursing. Although Nightingale had provided the emerging discipline with a relatively well-defined conceptualization of nursing, many aspects of this model were lost (or at least misplaced) in the increasing dominance of nursing by medicine. With this dominance came an increased reliance by many on an apprenticeship approach to basic "training" for nurses.

Peplau was among those dedicated to the development of nursing as a recognized professional discipline, focusing much of her effort on the development of a knowledge base to guide clinical practice. Peplau differentiates nursing and medicine: "physicians address themselves to within-person phenomena; to dysfunctions, deficits, defects and the life, in relation to the organism. They define the diseases of a person and prescribe treatment for them" (Riehl and Roy, p 14, 1980). In contrast to this definition of medicine, Peplau defines nursing as a "significant therapeutic interpersonal process which functions cooperatively with other human processes that make health possible for individuals" (Peplau, p 16, 1952).

To gain a perspective on the significance of the Peplau model of nursing, several sources were reviewed. According to Riehl and Roy (1974, 1980), Peplau provided an early attempt to analyze nursing action using an interpersonal theoretical framework, citing her book (Peplau, 1952) as a signficant contribution. The Nursing Development Conference Group (1973, 1979) recognized Peplau as a contributor to the development of nursing theory. She is credited by this group with formalizing the dependency theme between an individual who is sick and a nurse who is specially educated to recognize and respond to the need for help. Her contribution has been described by Gregg (1978) as excellence in teaching, consistency as a scholar, and creativity as a theoretician. She describes her "avid interest in the development of theory upon which clinical actions can be based" (p 120). Sills (1978) describes the impact of Peplau's contribution as responsible for a "second order change in the nursing culture" (p 124).

Placing the contribution in its chronological place in history, Peplau's interpersonal model initiates a move from an intrapsychic emphasis within psychiatric mental health nursing, and a dominant focus on physical care within general nursing to an interpersonal focus in both. Both Henderson and Orlando emphasize the interpersonal process, but both followed after Peplau with major publications including this emphasis. Once a contribution becomes a part of the public domain, it is difficult to estimate its impact on the larger society. Peplau's model, if it may be called that, is perhaps more of a middle range theory than a conceptual framework. The theory arises largely from clinical observations, and thus is inductive in nature.

BASIC CONSIDERATIONS

Definition of Nursing and Nursing Activity

Peplau's definition of nursing as "a maturing force and educative instrument" (Peplau, p 8, 1952) represents her view of the facilitative nature of the discipline. Its primary purpose is the application of scientific principles, particularly developmental principles, in facilitating human health. Peplau's earlier view of nursing as an applied science and as a process which aids patients to meet their own needs and recover from illness has been further developed. Her more recent conceptualization of nursing is that of a social and scientific force in the exploration and organization of factors relevant to the maintenance of health (Peplau, 1970, 1979).

Although Peplau describes nursing as a collaborative part of the health profession team, her model delineates a unique focus for nursing as resting in the reactions of the patient or client to circumstances of the illness or health problem. This focus was elaborated by Dorothy Gregg and cited by Peplau as "helping patients to gain intellectual and interpersonal competencies beyond that which they have at the point of illness. . . ." (Peplau, p 37, 1969). Nursing activity is, more specifically, depicted as six identified roles which the nurse assumes at various times during encounters with the patient. These roles are organized and operationalized through a four-phase interpersonal process. This process will be explained as a core component of Peplau's model. An elaboration of Peplau's definition of environment, person, and health provides background for explicating the ways in which nursing applies theoretical knowledge to function as a "maturing force" in individuals' lives.

Definition of Environment

The concept of environment is addressed primarily in reference to those external factors which are considered to be essential to human development. These include the presence of adults, secure economic status of the family, and a healthy prenatal environment (Peplau, p 163, 1952). More importantly, Peplau presents the interpersonal situations as environmental microcosms within which health is promoted. Interactions between person and family, child and parent, or patient and nurse are examples of this "interpersonal environment." Extension of the self into the community "and on into the ongoing stream of civilization" is required for the affirmation and fulfillment of human goals (Peplau, p 79, 1952). Cultural forces are other environmental factors by which societal values and mores significant to personality development are transmitted throughout life. Peplau also identifies the hospital as a physical and social environment and views it, as well as the nurse-patient interpersonal environment, as a primary responsibility of the nurse.

Definition of Person

The person, according to Peplau, is a developing self-system composed of biochemical, physiological, and interpersonal characteristics and needs. Development occurs as a result of interactions with significant others. Developmental tools are acquired as three sets of self-views emerge in development (Peplau, pp 35-37, 1979). These self-views influence the person's actions and range from those of which the person is consciously aware to those which are highly anxiety-producing and therefore repressed from conscious awareness. The self-views, to a large degree, consist of a synthesis of appraisals by others which have been introjected by the person.

The mature person is viewed as capable of meeting his or her own needs and integrating a variety of experiences. Human needs are organized hierarchically and give rise to transformations of energy into observable patterns of behavior designed to meet these needs. An individual's behavior patterns are partially determined by past developmental experiences, present contextual variables, and future expectations and goals. However, it is the person's perception of these factors that is particularly important in determining behavior.

The prototaxic, parataxic, and syntaxic modes of experiencing initially described by Sullivan (1952) affect perceptions of a given situation. The prototaxic mode refers to an experiencing characteristically found in infants which is limited to the present moment without relationship to the past or future. Parataxic thinking emerges as linkages between past, present, and future experiences develop and a familiar element can be identified to relate the three time dimensions. Persons in severe anxiety may have difficulty perceiving these linkages and the continuity between present and past events. The individual in the syntaxic mode is able to recognize the uniqueness of a given situation as well as its relationship to the past and future. As each of these modes becomes available, the person's ability to communicate with environmental resources and to problem-solve is enhanced.

Peplau (1952) states that persons live in an unstable equilibrium and have two basic goals, identified previously by Symonds (1946): self-maintenance and perpetuation of the species (p 79). All behavioral activities are purposeful and directed toward the reduction of anxiety generated from unmet needs and toward facilitating emergence of higher needs. These activities are based upon the interpersonal nature of the person. Human beings thrive on interpersonal relations. Such interpersonal experiences are significant both in facilitating solutions to anxiety situations for self maintenance, and in contributing to the development of additional anxiety in a person.

Anxiety As A Basic Concept

Anxiety is integral to Peplau's conceptualization of the person. It is an energy source inextricably related to human development from infancy to death and is required for biological and emotional growth (Peplau, 1963b). The theoretical frameworks of May (1960) and Sullivan (1952) are used to explicate this concept. "The self-system is an anti-anxiety system" (Peplau, p 36, 1979); directions for development are selected in reference to behaviors which prevent undue anxiety by meeting social expectations and biological needs.

Anxiety is produced when communications with others threaten the biological or psychological security of the individual (Peplau, 1963b). The presence and degree of anxiety experienced is inferred from the individual's patterns of behavior. A mild degree of anxiety heightens the person's sensitivity to the environment such that more information can be assimilated. The perceptual field becomes constricted as the degree of anxiety increases to the point where, in a state of panic, ability to test reality is seriously impaired. Identifiable behavior patterns emerge as the energy from varying degrees of anxiety is transformed. Some patterns, such as somatizing or withdrawing, are less effective in relieving anxiety than others which reflect more active attempts to problem-solve.

Debilitating behaviors are manifested in illness. In illness, and particularly during hospitalization, unmet needs and behavioral characteristics of less mature developmental stages are predominant. Illness is a time of regression and retreat to mobilize energy for use in reducing tension generated by unmet needs and conflicting goals.

Communication As A Basic Concept

Clear and supportive communication is a key element in a person's development. The significance attributed to communication in Peplau's (1952) model is reflected in her citation of Benjamin Whorf's theory that language mediates thought (Peplau, 1968). A person's thinking can be assessed and modified through communication with a significant other. For example, disturbed communication between a parent and a child can result in pathological modes of thought in the child (Peplau, p 77, 1979). Communication with others helps one to attend to and clarify one's perception of reality and to achieve a sense of understanding with another (Peplau, pp 290-294, 1952). This involves an awareness of nonverbal and verbal communication and the symbolic meaning behind these communications. It is one of the nurse's responsibilities to assess these factors and to influence the patient's communications in a manner that contributes to healthy modes of thought.

Definition of Health

Health is linked to the phenomenon of human development.The word "health" is a symbol that implies "forward movement of personality and other ongoing human processes in the direction of creative, constructive, productive, personal and community living" (Peplau, p 12, 1952). Human energy, derived from inevitable experiences of anxiety, can be transformed into either health-promoting or debilitating behaviors. Health-promoting behaviors as suggested by Peplau, are those which facilitate need satisfaction, self-awareness and meaningful integration of each of life's experiences, including illness. Health occurs when tension, due to unmet needs or unaccomplished developmental tasks, is relieved and energy is directed toward more mature goals.

Peplau's model places health and illness on a continuum. This health-illness continuum parallels Sullivan's (1947) conceptualization of a continuum of anxiety which Peplau (1952) depicts as ranging from pure euphoria to varying degrees of anxiety. The person's degree of health is related to the degree of anxiety experienced and the ability to transform this anxiety into productive, asymptomatic behavior. Health, then, is primarily based upon a reduction of anxiety.

Relationship of Basic Concepts to Health and Nursing

Reduction of anxiety and the resultant health state is dependent upon communications which facilitate an accurate perception of the problematic situation, identification and integration of related feelings and cognitions, and a reduction of anxiety through attainment of certain developmental skills. The experience of illness provides an opportunity for growth. Within this conceptualization, the patient can, through the nurse's intervention, develop communication skills and self-awareness that function to maintain a productive amount of anxiety in the self-system. The nurse's interventions are focused primarily upon the process of establishing and maintaining a trusting and goal-oriented relationship with the patient, that goal being the reduction of debilitating anxiety.

INTERNAL ANALYSIS

Underlying Assumptions

Peplau purports, for the most part, an inductive approach to model building. She seems to believe that theoretical concepts generally derive from empirical observations of patterns of phenomena, and that "nursing situations provide a field of observations from which unique nursing concepts can be derived and used for the improvement of the professional's work" (Peplau, p 36, 1969). Application of these concepts facilitates organization of observations and identification of potential solutions, and provides a structure for further exploration of the specific observed phenomena (Peplau, p 34, 1969).

Peplau also incorporates established knowledge in development of her nursing model. Peplau regards such knowledge as belonging to nursing when it facilitates selection and organization of a number of concepts into a larger component: 1) which delineates a serial ordering or a process of particular behaviors, i.e., Sullivan's (1952) outline of developmental tasks; 2) from which patient behavior can be understood and predicted; and 3) from which nursing interventions can be easily derived (Peplau, pp 34-36, 1969). Thus, Peplau includes in her model, as Ellis (1968) and Hardy (1974) advocate, a critical evaluation of knowledge from other areas for its relevance to nursing. Peplau's nursing model, then, represents the organization of selected concepts into a larger component which describes a sequence of behaviors that can be expected to occur in the nurse-patient relationship.

Central Components:
Definition and Relationships

There are four central components in Peplau's model: interpersonal process, nurse, patient, and anxiety. The interpersonal process is the central component of the model. It describes the method by which the nurse facilitates useful transformations of the patient's energy or anxiety. The interpersonal process represents the point at which the nurse and

patient interface in the interest of the patient's health. Characteristics of the nurse and patient are defined primarily in
reference to those which are considered relevant to the communication and changes that occur in human relationships,
and particularly in the nurse-patient relationship.

The interpersonal process is based upon a participatory
relationship between nurse and patient in which the nurse
governs the purpose and the process, and the patient controls the
content. The interpersonal process is operationally defined in
terms of four distinct phases: orientation, identification, exploitation, and resolution. Although it is described as having
distinct phases, overlapping is expected throughout the relationship. Phase one, orientation, has as its major focus helping patients
to become aware of the availability of and trust in the nurse's
abilities to participate effectively in his or her health care.
Identification, phase two, occurs when the nurse facilitates the
expression by the patient of whatever feelings are experienced,
and remains able to provide the nursing care needed. This expression without rejection permits the experiencing of illness
as an opportunity to reorient feelings and strengthen the positive
forces of the personality. A patient tends to respond to this
experience as an independent participant in the relationship
with the nurse, as an independent person in isolation from the
nurse, or as a dependent participant, helplessly dependent upon
the nurse.

The major working phase of the relationship is exploitation.
This third phase provides the situation in which the patient may
derive full value from the relationship in accordance with the
view or perception of the situation. This leads to the final phase,
resolution, during which the patient is gradually freed from the
identification with the helping professional. Resolution permits
the generation and strengthening of the ability to meet one's own
needs and to channel energy toward realization of potentialities
(Peplau, 1952). Thus, these four phases characterize a developmental process in which the nurse guides the patient from
dependent toward increasingly interdependent interactions with
the social environment.

The nurse is a component of the Peplau model; this is operationalized as a process in terms of any or all of six identified
roles. The first role, that of stranger, includes the sharing of respect and positive interest in the client. In the "stranger" role, the
nurse is at first non-personal and offers the same ordinary cour-
tesies that are accorded a guest when introduced into any new sit-

uation. These include acceptance of the person as she is and relating the patient as an emotionally able stranger unless there is evidence to support expectations of limitations in this area of functioning.

The second role is that of *resource* person. As resource person the nurse provides specific answers to questions which are usually formulated to address a larger problem. Answering these questions may lead to the emergence of more pertinent areas that require assistance. The third identified role, that of *teacher*, is viewed as a combination of all other roles. *Leadership*, the fourth identified role, is aimed toward the development of a democratic relationship, encouraging active participation of the patient/client in the direction of care. The nurse assumes the role of *surrogate* in situations that require resolution of existing interpersonal conflicts. Psychological age factors due to arrests in development or feelings reactivated through the experience of illness may demand the assumption of surrogate roles. Through this the nurse helps patients to learn that there are likenesses and differences between individuals, and by being herself assists with needed resolution of interpersonal conflicts.

The sixth role, that of *counselor*, is of major importance in all nurse-patient relationships. It is through this role that the nurse promotes experiences leading to health. Components of this role are: increasing a patient's awareness of conditions required for health and providing these when possible; identifying threats to health; and, facilitating learning through use of evolving interpersonal events. Through all of these roles, nursing behaviors of unconditional acceptance of the patient, self awareness, and an emotional neutrality are requisites (Peplau, 1952). These roles of the nurse describe mechanisms which the nurse uses throughout the interpersonal process. These roles imply, however, that the patient has the primary responsibility in reducing anxiety to a healthy level.

Peplau addresses the component, *patient*, primarily in terms of his or her experiences in illness with bound anxiety. Anxiety is manifested in various communications and affects the patient's ability to learn and function effectively. Peplau's assumption of human potentiality is evident in her model in that it depicts a direct relationship between the concepts of person and health; only the person can change the self and move toward health (Peplau, 1968). Interactions between the nurse and healthy person are of minor significance in Peplau's model, although in theory she conveys an awareness that the nurse has a role in health promotion as well as in reduction of anxiety (Figure 3.1, arrow D). Relationships among the central concepts of interpersonal process, nurse, patient, and anxiety are outlined in Figure 3.1.

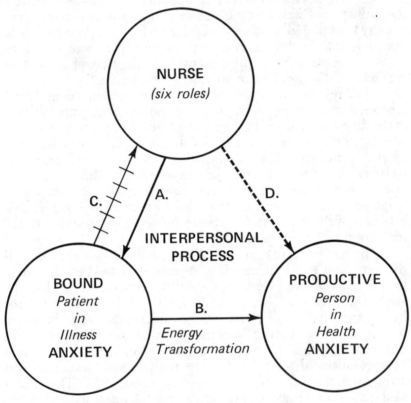

Figure 3.1. Peplau's Interpersonal Process Model of Nursing.

The nurse mediates the transformations of energy necessary for the patient's movement toward health. There is an indirect but vital relationship between nurse and eventual patient health (Peplau, p 83, 1952); that is, the nurse effects health outcomes through communication with the patient (Figure 3.1, arrow A). In this nurse-patient relationship, the patient is depicted as a recipient of the effects of the interpersonal process and has little effect upon the nurse. Peplau recommends that the nurse, as part of the patient's interpersonal environment, maintain a neutral emotional position and resist being influenced by the patient (Figure 3.1, arrow C). However, the potential effect of the patient upon the nurse is acknowledged in Peplau's admonition for nurses to understand themselves and their reactions to the patient. In general, minimal emphasis is given to the patient's effect upon the physical or social factors in the environment that are encountered during illness. Affecting the environment in service of the patient's health is more the responsibility of the nurse than the patient.

Anxiety As A Pivotal Concept In Peplau's Model

There is a direct relationship between anxiety and illness. In illness, energy from anxiety needed for growth is instead bound in non-healthy symptoms such as headache, unexplained fever, or suicidal ideation (Peplau, p 100, 1952). A major goal of nursing is to assess the degree of anxiety existing in a patient's life, the ways in which it is communicated by both patient and nurse, its effects upon the patient's ability to learn and maintain healthy behavior patterns, and to implement strategies which effectively reduce debilitating levels of anxiety. The nurse, through interpersonal interaction with the patient, facilitates the patient's ability to transform symptom-bound energy into problem-solving energy. The resulting reduction in anxiety moves the patient toward health (Figure 3.1, arrow B).

Internal Consistency

Peplau's model is consistent with her definition of nursing as an "educative instrument" (Peplau, 1952; 1963a; 1979). The interpersonal process is organized around the patient learning about himself or herself, the health problem, and healthy attitudes and practices. This learning process involves "educing"—a root of the word "education"—from the patient thoughts and feelings needed to initiate change and problem-solving activities (Peplau, p 275, 1968). Moreover, Peplau's assumption that only the individual can change himself or herself is elucidated in her emphasis upon the nurse as a facilitator as well as educator in the interpersonal relationship.

Peplau's explication of the interpersonal process is adequate as defined by Hardy (1974). The four phases of the interpersonal process provide an operational definition of nursing activity. The phases depict a logical progression of the nurse-patient relationship and are consistent with the developmental theories upon which they are based. In particular, the psychological tasks described by Sullivan (1952) of learning to trust, to set realistic limits, to gain self-identity, and to participate and validate within a community of others, are incorporated into the definitions and purposes of Peplau's phases of orientation, exploitation, implementation, and resolution (Peplau, pp 3-42, 161-259, 1952; Peplau, pp 1-7, 1969).

Further analysis of Peplau's (1952) model reveals some lack of consistency in her meanings of the concept person, and the relationship between nurse and patient. According to Hardy (1974), the meanings attributed to the basic concepts and the logic by which they are related are included as criteria for internal consistency. Peplau's model depicts a goal of human activity as striving toward a sense of equilibrium through self-maintenance and tension-reducing activities. Yet, similar to Maslow, Peplau explicates the person's limitless potential for learning and for the transformation of energy to accomplish increasingly mature goals. This formulation is more compatible with the later-developed open system view. Thus, the definition of person is not consistent throughout the model and limits operational adequacy.

What initially appears to be an inconsistency in Peplau's model may instead be an early attempt to reformulate existing closed-system theories of human development in a way that would account for the nursing perspective of the person as interdependent with the environment and capable of employing available resources to regain health and further development. Peplau's incorporation of the interpersonal process in her model initiates a shift in emphasis from an intrapsychic to an interpersonal perspective of human development and well-being. The environment, at least in terms of other human beings and their behaviors and feelings, has been increasingly identified as a significant factor in health and development.

Peplau's early model emphasizes the importance of the nurse maintaining an objective and a neutral or nonjudgmental stance in relationships with patients. This view is interpreted as Peplau's appreciation for and understanding of the significant difference between friendships and therapeutic relationships, wherein the latter relationship exists primarily for the needs of the patient rather than both parties. Although the emphasis attributed to the nurse's objectivity in Peplau's early model is not entirely consistent with the more recent open-system theories regarding the inevitable mutuality of exchange between the person and environment, it is more consistent with the views prevalent when Peplau was developing her model.

Peplau's (1952) model postulates a directional relationship between person and environment wherein the environment stimulates emergency of needs in the person. Moreover, the environment, in terms of its cultural forces, interacts with the individual's biological processes in determining personality characteristics. The model, however, does not indicate a reciprocity between person and environment. Although her model attests to the importance of the environment, it does not explicitly identify ways by which the patient can modify the environment to reduce debilitating anxiety. This may be viewed to limit the usefulness of the model.

Because Peplau was committed to theory-based nursing practice at a time when nursing theory development was relatively unknown, it is understood that Peplau could not disregard the reductionistic conceptualizations extant during the development of her model. Theories that were available for integration into her model at that time depicted human behavior within the perspectives of biologically-based psychoanalytic theory, stimulus-response models, and closed-system notions of tension-reduction and equilibrium maintenance. Peplau utilized concepts from these theories in constructing a conceptual model for psychodynamic nursing.

Persons seeking health care were approached in terms of their illness rather than their inherent potentialities. The resulting focus upon the ill person and ways to reduce anxiety, although it is congruent with the thinking at that time, limits the usefulness of Peplau's model in reference to the nurse's role with the healthy person. It is remarkable, although somewhat internally inconsistent, that Peplau also integrated within her psychodynamic model broad nursing perspectives regarding the significance of interpersonal processes and social factors, ongoing energy transformation, the patient's unlimited potential for health, and the facilitative role of the nurse.

It is important to note that Peplau's later writings clearly indicate a conceptual movement away from some of the earlier reductionistic principles in a way that is not entirely consistent with theoretical ideas of her 1952 model of nursing. For example, Peplau's (1963a) exposition on the concept of learning implies a reconceptualization of the learning principles of Miller and Dollard (1941) which she initially used as a theoretical base for explicating phases of the interpersonal process (Peplau, p 34, 1952).

The patient, in her revised model, is conceptualized as interdependent with the environment to a greater degree and capable of initiating change, rather than as a "follower" of the nurse as "leader." Still other writings reflect an increasing focus upon the importance of the social significance of environment in health and of nursing's role in terms of health maintenance rather than recovery from illness (Peplau, 1970). These ideas are more consistent with contemporary views of nursing than they are with the reductionistic and medically-oriented views of the patient.

EXTERNAL ANALYSIS

Nursing Research

Peplau postulated several questions that are topics of research today. Her interpersonal model operationalized concepts which can be used in exploring the effectiveness of the nursing process in predicting patient behavior. One concern expressed by Peplau (1952) was whether or not the nursing process facilitated need satisfaction and enhanced growth of the patient (p 10). The roles and interpersonal process provide structure that can be used to study the movement of the patient from a dependent to independent to interdependent relationship with the nurse, rather than focus research on the dependency of the patient upon the helper.

Peplau (1952) also indicated the need to explore the meaning of health and the conditions which promote physical and social well-being (p 11). Her model, which incorporated such ideas as energy transformation and the forward movement of development, addresses health in somewhat abstract terms. Operationalizations of the concept of health would be necessary before such an exploration could occur. However, her model provides a theoretical framework for research about health (anxiety reduction), particularly mental health, in that it has defined health and movement toward health in reference to a more or less coherent synthesis of theories about communication, learning, anxiety, and human development.

Peplau is explicit in stating the importance of theoretically based nursing practice (1969; 1970). Her statements are supportive of theory-building research to the extent that she indicates the need for reformulation of theories from other disciplines. However, her model (1952) does not clearly differentiate between methodology for practice and methodology appropriate for the testing of principles upon which practice is based. It is implied that data collected within the interpersonal process can be used in theory testing as well as in assessment of the patient. Although research issues conceptualized from within a nursing perspective are needed, using data collected for clinical purposes for research is not a recommended approach to theory-building (Walker, 1971). Peplau's quest for a sound theoretical base for all nursing activity continues to be a major incentive for sound nursing research, and it will become a reality as more nurses acquire sophistication in research strategies.

Nursing Education

Peplau contributed significantly to moving the nursing profession into graduate education (Gregg, 1978). Her model has been used extensively in educating both undergraduate and graduate nursing students about a major component of nursing activities—the interpersonal relationship. In particular, it has provided theoretically based knowledge for nursing specialization in psychiatric settings wherein the one-to-one relationship is the primary methodology for nursing.

Nursing Practice

Peplau's model has served as a conceptual framework for psychodynamic nursing since 1952 and continues to be a relevant model for nursing psychotherapy today (Peplau, 1952, 1979; Sills, 1977, 1978). It provides clear direction to nursing practice through the six roles and the four phases of the interpersonal process. Nursing practitioners use these to clarify nursing's focus in health care as well as to facilitate collaboration with other health care professionals and the patient.

In particular, the four phases of the nurse-patient relationship presented earlier are clearly defined; Peplau has operationalized these phases to facilitate their application in a wide variety of nurse-patient settings, particularly when the focus is mental health. Although the phases are abstract concepts, Peplau's model delineates observable, behavioral indicators of characteristics of each phase (Peplau, 1952, 1969).

In addition, Peplau's regard for effective communication between nurse and patient is applicable to nursing practice. An understanding of verbal and nonverbal communication of both the nurse and patient are considered basic to the nursing process. Through various communication skills, the nurse can: convey interest and concern to the patient; clarify and validate assumptions about the patient; help the patient formulate meaning of the identified problems; and, generally guide the patient in transforming anxiety-based energy to solve the problems.

Investigative interviewing is a type of communication used by the nurse to determine the self views that are operative in a patient's life. Through this process, the nurse works to uncover latent or unused capacities of the patient and to help the patient realize and implement them in his or her recovery. Peplau also addresses the significance of communication skills in the development of nursing as a profession. She encourages a sharing, clarifying, and validating of ideas in the careful selection of nursing concepts that are meaningful to both the culture and its need for nursing services, and to nurses providing the services (Peplau, p 4-5, 290-291, 1952).

The following example demonstrates the applicability of Peplau's model to nursing practice. Tom was a sixteen year-old boy who had recently experienced a series of stresses within his family, including the death of his father. He had become increasingly withdrawn and depressed and had on several occasions asked his mother if she would be terribly upset if he were to die too. He entered the nurse's office on his first visit to the clinic with a mixed look of relief and reluctance, and hurriedly told the nurse that he was coming to see her only long enough to rid himself of his "rotten feelings."

It was an important aspect of the orientation phase of their relationship that Tom felt some need to visit the nurse regularly since the relationship was one in which both parties have a responsibility to participate. The nurse assumed several roles throughout the initial sessions. As stranger, she encouraged him to ask questions, to familiarize himself with the purpose and arrangement of the clinic and her professional qualifications, and generally to feel comfortable in the new situation. As counselor she listened actively to Tom's perception of his problems and helped him to identify and clarify relevant issues.

The nurse became less of a stranger to Tom as his initial anxiety was transformed into trust in their relationship and as he began to identify the nurse as a caring and capable individual. These characteristics of the relationship mark the second phase, identification. During this phase, Tom expressed ambivalent feelings toward the nurse. Often he wanted to cry and lay all of his feelings and pain before her, but his desire to do this would make him angry at feeling so dependent. At times, he would test his relationship and dependency upon the nurse by arriving late to their appointment or refusing to talk about his problems. Throughout this phase the nurse utilized both the surrogate and leadership roles with Tom. She would emphasize the surrogate role when she conveyed needed acceptance and nurturance to Tom either as he expressed his "shameful" thoughts or during his angry silences. As a leader, the nurse would suggest possible meanings behind his feelings, validate her interpretations with him, and when necessary, direct the topic of their communications or redefine the purpose of their relationship.

During the phase of exploitation, Tom and the nurse used the strength of their relationship to discuss Tom's problems and to identify ways in which Tom's energy could be more profitably used in his schoolwork and in family and social relationships. The nurse's role of teacher became particularly salient during this phase.

Tom used his relationship with the nurse to explore meanings of some of his and other family members' grieving behaviors in response to his father's death. The exploitation phase of the relationship also was a time for confronting and clarifying Tom's prototaxic distortions from the earlier phases of the relationship in which he responded to the nurse as a parent-like figure who demanded dependence and obedience. These developmental issues of adolescence as well as the more serious problems were discussed and brought closer to resolution. Tom had opportunities to test out his learnings in everyday situations and to return at the next session to evaluate the experience with the nurse. Thus, a variety of issues were exploited to help Tom redirect energy toward the more productive tasks of his developmental level.

As new goals were identified, Tom began to realize that he had learned from the nurse all he could at that time. He was then ready to terminate the relationship. He compared his feelings during termination with those related to his father's death: those of hurt, anger, and sadness. Tom was, however, able to recognize and accept the feelings, and then to release his identification with the nurse. Thus, Tom moved from a dependence upon the nurse, through rebellious attempts at independence, to the achievement of an interdependent relationship. As a result of this interpersonal relationship with the nurse, Tom learned how to acknowledge and cherish the good feelings of a terminated relationship and yet feel free and secure enough as an individual to anticipate the benefits and risks of future relationships.

SUMMARY

Peplau has developed a nursing model that is useful in a variety of nursing contexts in which the nurse is engaged in a therapeutic relationship with a patient. The model is not complex, as defined by Ellis (1968), and it relates a limited number of concepts in an understandable way. It may be described as a "practice-oriented" model, applicable to clinical practice; thus, it holds one of the prime characteristics of significance for nursing (Ellis, p 220, 1968; Jacox, 1974). Although the components and relationships within Peplau's model are not explicit enough to meet criteria for a theory (Hardy, 1974), her concepts of interpersonal process, anxiety, and communication define broad areas which continue to be relevant to current nursing practice and research.

Peplau has been exemplary in her approach to using theories originating in other disciplines in model building. Her ideas reflect a process of reformulating existing theories from such persons as Maslow (1943) and Sullivan (1947) in such a way that the theories were compatible with and relevant to the empirical world of nursing activity. These reformulations resulted primarily in the development of Peplau's interpersonal process for nursing. Her process of reformulation becomes evident as one studies the nearly thirty years of her published works. Peplau has not limited herself to closed-system views of the patient; instead, she has acknowledged the purposeful, affective behavior and inherent potential for development. Peplau's model interfaces with the shift in paradigms from the intrapsychic to the interpersonal approach in the therapeutic relationship.

Most important, perhaps, is Peplau's contribution to the fulfillment of Nightingale's vision for knowledge-based nursing practice. Knowledge, whether from another discipline and reformulated, or originated by nurses, can play a role in the development of nursing theories (Ellis, 1968). Peplau's model provided nursing with a meaningful method of self-directed practice at a time when medicine dominated the health-care field. Although initially controversial, the interpersonal process has, over the years, been integrated into both nursing practice and education.

REFERENCES

Ellis R: Characteristics of significant theories. Nursing Research, Vol 17, No 3, pp 217-222, 1968

Gregg DE: Hildegard E. Peplau: her contributions. Perspective in Psychiatric Care, Vol 16, No 3, pp 118-121, 1978

Hardy ME: Theories: components, development, evaluation. Nursing Research, Vol 23, No 2, pp 188-187, 1974

Jacox A: Theory construction in nursing. Nursing Research, Vol 23, No 1, pp 4-12, 1974

Maslow AH: A theory of human motivation. Psychological Review, Vol 58, pp 378-396, July 1943

May R: The Meaning of Anxiety. The Ronald Press Co., New York, 1950

Miller NE, Dollard J: Social Learning and Imitation. Yale University Press, New Haven, Connecticut, 1941

Nursing Development Conference Group: Concept Formalization in Nursing: Process and Product. Little, Brown & Co., Boston, Massachusetts, 1973

Nursing Development Conference Group: Concept Formalization in Nursing: Process and Product, 2nd ed. Little, Brown & Co., Boston, Massachusetts, 1979

Peplau HE: Interpersonal Relations in Nursing. G. P. Putnam's Sons, New York, 1952

Peplau HE: Process and concept of learning. In Burd SF, Marshall MA (eds): Some Clinical Approaches to Psychiatric Nursing, Macmillan, New York, 1963a

Peplau HE: A working definition of anxiety. In Burd SF, Marshall MA (eds): Some Clinical Approaches to Psychiatric Nursing, Macmillan, New York, 1963b

Peplau HE: Psychotherapeutic strategies. Perspectives in Psychiatric Care, Vol 6, No 6, pp 264-278, 1968

Peplau HE: Theory: the professional dimension. In Norris C (ed): Proceedings of the First Nursing Theory Conference, University of Kansas Medical Center, Department of Nursing Education, March 21-28, 1969

Peplau HE: ANA's new executive director states her views. American Journal of Nursing, Vol 70, No 1, pp 84-88, 1970

Peplau HE: The Psychotherapy of Hildegard E. Peplau, WE Field (ed). PSF Productions, New Braunfels, Texas, 1979

Riehl, JP, Roy C: Conceptual Models for Nursing Practice. Appleton-Century-Crofts, New York, 1974

Riehl, JP, Roy C: Conceptual Models for Nursing Practice, 2nd ed. Appleton-Century-Crofts, New York, 1980

Sills GM: Research in the field of psychiatric nursing 1952-1977. Nursing Research, Vol 26, No 3, pp 281-287, 1977

Sills GM: Hildegard E. Peplau: leader, practitioner, academician, scholar, and theorist. Perspectives in Psychiatric Care, Vol 16, No 3, pp 122-128, 1978

Sullivan HS: Conceptions of Modern Psychiatry. William Alanson White Psychiatric Foundation, Washington, D.C., 1947

Sullivan HS: The Interpersonal Theory of Psychiatry. W. W. Norton &
    Co., Inc., New York, 1952
Symonds P: The Dynamics of Human Adjustment. Appleton-Century-
    Crofts, Inc., New York, 1946
Walker LO: Toward a clearer understanding of the concept of nursing
    theory. Nursing Research, Vol 28, No 5, pp 428-434, 1971

4

IDA ORLANDO'S
MODEL OF NURSING

Claire M. Andrews

INTRODUCTION

Orlando's impetus to develop her model was recognition that inadequate nursing care existed and the subsequent desire for an optimal level of nursing care (Orlando, 1961, 1972; Pelletier, 1967). Orlando advocated deliberative nursing care which is distinct from other health professions. She was one of the first to recognize the critical element of patient validation of needs and likewise validation as to whether the nurses' actions were successful in helping the patient. Orlando's model was the first to emphasize patient participation in planning care and in patient feedback. In this discussion, it is recognized that Orlando's model is an early one and not therefore as fully developed as later nursing models.

In 1954 the National Institute of Mental Health of the United States Public Health Service awarded the Yale University School of Nursing a project grant. At the end of the four year project and at the time her first book was published, Orlando was Director of the Graduate Program at Yale in Mental Health and Psychiatric Nursing. Her book, *The Dynamic Nurse-Patient Relationship*, (Orlando, 1961) contained in part the findings from the NIMH study. The book dealt with the subject matter and process for integrating mental health principles into a basic nursing curriculum. In essence, a secondary purpose of the book was to offer the professional nursing student a model of effective nursing practice.

Orlando emphasizes similar aspects of professional nursing care in a later article and book (Orlando, 1967, 1972). In her article (Pelletier, 1967) she extends the model for nurses as well as for collaborative staff relationships. At the time of Orlando's second book, *The Discipline and Teaching of Nursing Process* (1972), she was a clinical nursing consultant at a private psychiatric hospital. This work was a continuation of her first endeavors; i.e., the nursing model contained in *The Dynamic Nurse-Patient Relationship* was further developed, implemented, and evaluated and the results comprised the contents of the book. In this latter work the emphasis is on the verbal form of a nursing process that is effective in patient, staff, and supervisor contacts.

Nursing and society influenced Orlando's thinking regarding her model in the years prior to the initiation of the project grant as well as during the period while she was at Yale. In the post World War II years, there was a diligent "return to normalcy" effort in our society. Also during that time there was a slowly increasing recognition and respect for the individual. Whether a result of post-war influences or not, nursing diligently moved toward higher education in and autonomy of the nursing profession. The nursing literature from that time on gave evidence of a growing appreciation and desire for quality nursing care as educated nurses recognized the potential for nursing.

In 1952, Hildegarde Peplau's book, *Interpersonal Relations in Nursing*, was published. Peplau was a psychiatric nurse, and her work was almost certain to have influenced Orlando's model. Also in the post-war period, a number of nurses had the opportunity to share ideas, and concerns relevent to nursing developed during attendance at institutions of higher education. Orlando specifically identified three areas with which the nursing profession was concerned at the time: nurse-patient relationships, the nurse's professional role, and the identity and development of knowledge which is distinctly nursing. Also an influence was Wiedenbach's work in maternity nursing.

Orlando and Wiedenbach were both at Yale. Orlando incorporated many maternity examples into her book. There are certain similarities in their ideas; e.g., Wiedenbach's model focuses on comfort and capability and Orlando's model deals with comfort and sense of adequacy.

ANALYSIS OF BASIC CONSIDERATIONS

Orlando describes nursing knowledge as "related to people, their environment and their health" (Orlando, p 1, 1961). She defines these concepts within the framework of her model of nursing. She does not fully develop or refine the concepts of person, health, or environment. Orlando perceives these concepts as properties characteristic of nursing and uses them as she explicates her concept of nursing. Thus their meanings are understood within the framework of her nursing model.

Person

Orlando conceptualizes person as a "behaving human organism." In her view, neither nursing knowledge or practice deals with all persons but rather is concerned with those under medical supervision or treatment, because nursing as a profession has traditionally aligned itself with the practice of medicine (Orlando, p 5, 1961). Orlando views medicine as "that art and science which deals with and is responsible for the prevention and treatment of disease" (Orlando, p 5, 1961).

Whatever help patients may require for their needs to be met is, according to Orlando, the responsibility of the nurse (Orlando, p 5, 1961). Nurses provide physical and mental comfort through some mode of interaction. The importance of the nurse being able to recognize a person's health needs is evident. However, the nurse must discriminate further because those needs that patients can meet comfortably on their own are not of professional concern to the nurse (Orlando, p 6, 1961). It then becomes imperative, according to Orlando, that the nurse learn to understand patients and their needs, recognizing the individuality of a person and consequent unique situations. It is also evident that the nurse must recognize the person's abilities and strengths.

Environment

Orlando's model "has been successfully applied in the nursing of patients with medical, surgical, obstetric and psychiatric conditions and is applicable to the nursing of adults and children whether in the home, hospital or clinic"(p viii). The actual nursing situations that Orlando discusses occur in the hospital, but the application of her model needs a nurse and a patient and is not limited by a place. The environment becomes important because it affects the immediate and individual character of a nursing situation (Orlando, p 1, 1961). The nurse, according to Orlando, must work with the patient in a specific time and place, and thus what the nurse observes, and how the nurse acts in regard to this context, is important to it (Orlando, p 1, 1961). A nurse acts for the benefit of a patient so that nursing action may be taken to change the immediate environment (Orlando, p 60, 1961).

Health

Orlando proposes that the nurse achieves her purpose when she contributes to the mental and physical health of the patient (Orlando, p 9, 1961). She interchanges the word health with the word comfort, i.e., mental and physical comfort. Orlando also relates that in helping patients, the nurse positively influences their sense of adequacy or well-being. The help received is also considered to have a cumulative value as it contributes individuals' adequacy in taking better care of themselves (Orlando, p 9, 1961). In brief, Orlando's concept of health seems to deal with comfort, adequacy, and well-being.

Nursing

Orlando does not explicitly define the concept of nursing. She does, however, explain the facets of nursing in order to provide an understanding of the concept of nursing. These facets include nursing knowledge, the focus and purpose of nursing, the responsibility of nurses, and general description of nursing practice. The latter also provides a description of the interrelationships between the basic concepts.

Nursing knowledge is based on concepts and principles from the basic and applied sciences and medical specialties as well as mental and public health concepts (Orlando, p 1, 1961).The immediate and individual character of the nursing situation directed at helping the patient distinguishes these concepts and principles as nursing (Orlando, p 1, 1961). Other fields of theory have their own distinct aims and responsibilities (Orlando, p 3, 1961). Knowledge from other fields of practice does not guide nursing practice but can be used as a resource upon which the nurse can draw (Orlando, p 3, 1961). In this model, the broader the nurse's knowledge base, the greater the resources upon which she can draw to help the patient (Orlando, p 3, 1961).

Orlando proposes that for effective nursing care, the exclusive focus of nursing is the patient and the patient's needs. According to Orlando, "*the purpose of professional nursing is to supply the help a patient requires in order for his needs to be met*" (Orlando, p 8, 1961). Inherent in this definition is what Orlando refers to as a rudimentary concept of nursing; namely, "any individual nurses another when he carries, whole or in part, the burden of responsibility for what the person cannot yet or can no longer do alone" (Orlando, p 5, 1961). Orlando maintains, then, that the responsibility of a nurse is to help patients meet their needs, i e., to provide for their physical and mental comfort while they are undergoing some form of medical treatment or supervision. The success of treatment of preventive measures rests on the patient's own capacity to use them (Orlando, p 23, 1961).

Specifically, the nurse assumes the responsibility for seeking out and obviating impediments to the patient's mental and physical comfort (Orlando, p 9, 1961). In doing so the nurse helps the patient avoid or alleviate the distress of unmet needs (Orlando, p 6, 1961). A person who is ill is likely to have his/her sense of adequacy or well-being disrupted (Orlando, p vii, 1961), and the nurse helps the patient maintain or retain the patient's sense of adequacy or well-being in stressful situations associated with the patient's illness. In general, the nurse provides help when the patient's distress stems from physical limitations, adverse reactions to the setting, and experiences which prevent the patient from communicating his/her needs (Orlando, p 11, 1961). By recognizing the nature of the patient's distress and the need for help, the nurse can identify her professional function as she provides for the patient's mental and physical comfort.

The nurse must help meet the patient's need directly or indirectly by calling upon others for help. The nurse meets the need indirectly when she directs non-professional personnel to carry out activities which meet the patient's needs, or when she/he helps the patient obtain the services of a person, agency, or resource by which his/her need can be met (Orlando, p 8, 1961). The nurse meets the patient's need directly in a nursing situation when a patient is unable to meet his/her own need (Orlando, p 8, 1961). A nursing situation involves the behavior of the patient, the reaction of the nurse, and the nursing actions designed for the patient's benefit. The nursing process is the interaction of those elements with each other (Orlando, p 36, 1981).

What a nurse says or does is the exclusive mode through which a nurse serves a patient. Since the patient and nurse are both people, they interact and a process occurs between them (Orlando, p 6, 1961). According to Orlando, learning to understand what is happening between oneself and the patient is the central core of the nurse's practice; this also comprises the basic framework for practice. To meet the patient's needs, the nurse first initiates a process of helping the patient express the specific meaning of the patient's behavior to ascertain the patient's distress (Orlando, p 29, 1961). This aspect of nursing practice is especially important because "people are ambivalent in relation to their dependency needs" (Orlando, p 24, 1961). Secondly, the nurse helps the patient explore the distress in order to ascertain the help that the patient requires so that the patient's distress may be relieved (Orlando, p 29, 1961). A deliberative nursing process involves continuous reflection as the nurse tries to understand the meaning of the behavior to the patient. The nurse also attempts to discern what the patient needs from the nurse in order to be helped (Orlando, p 67, 1961).

The nurse must explore how the patient is affected by what the nurse says or does. The nurse cannot assume that any aspect of her/his reaction to the patient is correct, helpful, or appropriate until the validity of it has been checked with the patient (Orlando, p 56, 1961). "Understanding how practices help or do not help the patient is the material out of which the nurse develops and improves her knowledge and skill in practice" (Orlando, p 6, 1961). This process allows for the unique character of any nurse-patient situation (Orlando, p 67, 1961).

Nursing activity does not always meet patients' needs either because the needs are of no concern or because nursing activities are automatic. Needs that patients can meet comfortably on their own are not of any professional concern to the nurse (Orlando, p 6, 1961). A nurse's activity is professional only when it deliberatively achieves the purpose of helping the patient (Orlando, p 7, 1961). If the nursing activity is not deliberative, then it is automatic, i.e., the activities are carried out without exploration of the patient's need or consideration of how the nursing activity affects the patient (Orlando, p 65, 1961). Although any nursing activity can be considered automatic, specific examples include routines of patient care (food service, morning care, etc.), routines which protect the interests and safety of the patient (siderails, restricting visitors, isolation techniques, etc.), and routines which protect the organization (permission slips, release signatures, etc.) (Orlando, p 85, 1961). Although these are automatic activities, the nurse must be sure of the effect they have on the patient. Even though routines of care, medical orders, and activities are based on health principles and are intended to help the patient, deliberation is needed to determine whether the activity achieves its purpose and whether the patient is helped by it (Orlando, p 60, 1961).

Orlando is aware that the organization of nursing in some settings requires the nurse to carry out activities unrelated to the professional task. She also asserts that preoccupation with other tasks decreases the nurse's freedom to help the patient (Orlando, p 70, 1961).

INTERNAL ANALYSIS AND EVALUATION

Assumptions

Orlando has both implicit and explicit assumptions which support her model of nursing. Assumptions are abstract, in that they are not themselves reality but help structure the theory, thereby proposing guides and controls in shaping reality (Dickoff & James, 1968). Therefore, when considering certain extenuating circumstances, these assumptions can be reshaped in the continuing development of the theory.

In the following section several assumptions are identified. The first assumption to be considered is that nursing is distinct from other scientific fields. An explanation regarding this assumption was previously presented in the explanation of nursing and practice. The distinction of what is uniquely nursing is made primarily with the application of principles from other fields.

Another assumption Orlando makes is that persons are behaving human organisms. This assumption is necessary for implementing the nursing process as Orlando describes it. Orlando describes primarily verbal behavior which is consistent with this assumption, in addition to recognizing other forms of behavior. In the case of an infant, a fetus, or an adult whose behavior is difficult to assess, the nurse, according to Orlando, does (or "behaves") for patients what they can no longer do or have not yet been able to do for themselves. The nurse avoids or obviates the distress of unmet needs which may arise from physical limitations. According to Hardy (1974), "behaving" may be termed a primitive or undefined concept.

The next assumption to be considered is that nursing is aligned with medicine, to the extent that nursing responsibility is only to those undergoing medical treatment or supervision. Essentially this assumption is concerned with Orlando's concept of patient. Although there is consistency with this approach throughout her model, this reliance upon medical relationship can be considered a limitation to nursing practice. In other words, nurses could not nurse anyone who is not the patient of a physician. This assumption ties nurses and nursing to medical systems and institutions, and thus restricts the scope of persons, health, and environments that concern nurses and nursing. This assumption is not really necessary for the overall application of Orlando's model; it could be adapted by removing the word "only." This adaptation would extend and broaden the model to apply to those persons for whom the nurse provides care.

The next assumption is that there is a clear distinction between medical management (which deals with the treatment and prevention of disease) and nursing management (which deals with the way patients would manage their own affairs and their own contacts if they were able to do so). Again this is consistent with Orlando's concept of patient and is helpful in directing nursing care. If the assumption were interpreted loosely and/or with a broadened concept of patient, the scope of nursing practice would be dramatically extended. This assumption is valuable for nursing because it recognizes nursing as an autonomous profession. Orlando supports this assumption in small but very important ways; e.g., physicians do not write orders for nurses, but for patients, and nurses do for patients what they (patients) cannot do for themselves. There is some inconsistency in Orlando's model. Specifically, the terms treatment and prevention are introduced as concepts for medical management, yet some nursing activities can be interpreted as both treatment and prevention. Also, if nurses include prevention as part of their practice, in some cases the concept of person would necessarily be extended beyond medical patients.

Another assumption made by Orlando is that the nurse is concerned only with those needs that patients cannot meet comfortably on their own. This assumption places a boundary upon nursing's responsibility. However, it does evoke a question when considering the nursing process as described by Orlando: should nurses not address or at least initiate the nursing process to determine patients' needs, what patients are doing to meet their needs, or whether, in fact, patients are attempting to meet their needs?

Another assumption is that nursing interaction is beneficial and does not add to the distress of the patient. This may not always be the case. For example, in certain instances there might be an increase in distress before a decrease in distress occurs. For example, when receiving an injection, the distress with regards to having the injection occurs, but once the injection is over, the patient may have a sense of well-being as a result of the procedure. Also there might be an immediate change for the better in the patient's condition.

Central Components

Orlando's model, like other nursing models, contains concepts or components which are basic to all nursing theory as well as concepts which are specific to Orlando. An example of both types of concepts are these: patient, need, interaction, validation, health, improvement, and nursing.

One central concept of this model as well as others is that of the patient. Orlando considers a patient to be "a behaving human organism"—her definition of person. A patient is someone undergoing some form of medical treatment or supervision (Orlando, p 5, 1961). In terms of the meaning attributed to patient there may be some question of intersubjectivity (Hardy, 1974; Reynolds, 1971). Some would dispute the definition as being restricted by the consideration of "medicine." Undoubtedly Orlando's definition of patient stems from the position of nursing with relation to medicine at the time that the book was first written.

In recent years, with expanding roles for nurses, the definition of Orlando's concept of patient may be questioned; also, her definition might be expanded to mean all recipients of nursing care.

Another central component is need. Orlando's definition is "... *need is situationally defined as a requirement of the patient which, if supplied, relieves or diminishes his immediate distress or improves his immediate sense of adequacy or well being*" (Orlando, p 5, 1961). According to Hardy (1974), this is acceptable as a theoretical definition because it gives meaning to a term in context of the theory and allows for validity to be assessed.

If patients can meet their needs on their own, the nurse, according to Orlando, would not be concerned with the needs (Orlando, p 6, 1961). The nurse is responsible for helping the patient avoid or alleviate the distress of unmet needs (Orlando, p 6, 1961). In order for the nurse to recognize met and unmet needs, the nurse must understand the kinds of experiences which may distress patients (Orlando, p 6, 1961). According to Orlando, patients generally require help when their distresses stem from physical limitations, adverse reactions to the setting, and experiences which prevent patients from communicating their needs (Orlando, p 11, 1961). Without Orlando's concept of patient, her definition of need would be difficult to understand. The concept of patient gives considerable definition to the concept of need. One concern with Orlando's definiton of need is the use of the term immediate. This term allows for great consistency in her theory, e.g., in relation to improvement as a central component. The concern with the term "immediate" is that it does not account for long-term needs.

Another component of the model is that of interaction. The elements of interaction are the patient's behavior and nurse's action and reaction (Orlando, p 36, 1961). In other words, interaction involves what happens as well as how it happens in relation to the process of helping the patient. Nursing interaction involves recognition of the distinction between generally useful activities and specific ones that meet the needs of the patient. The concept of interaction is emphasized by Orlando, possibly to the detriment of her model. Orlando seems to equate interaction with the nursing process she describes. In the numerous illustrations of nursing situations, Orlando is both very general and very specific as to descriptions of interactions. The meaning of this concept thus needs refinement in the sense that the concept is empirically and theoretically adequate but operational adequacy is questioned. The nursing process is illustrated as a verbal process, when in fact it becomes apparent that Orlando does not intend to place a limitation on the scope of the concept of interaction. Orlando did attempt to refine the term interaction, particularly as it relates to a verbal process in her other words (Orlando, 1972; Pelletier, 1967). Her second book is the result of a research study related to the verbal form of interaction.

Health seems to be another central component in Orlando's model. Whether this is a central component is questioned primarily because of its indirect inclusion into the definition of need. Orlando equates physical and mental health to a sense of adequacy or well-being, and to physical and mental comfort. Orlando does not directly state that these terms are equated, but does so indirectly by interchanging the terms at critical points. Health is part of the measured outcome of nursing action. For this reason, a more refined operational definition of health would have been valuable.

Another term used by Orlando is that of improvement. Improvement is defined *"to grow better, to turn to profit, to use to advantage"* (Orlando, p 6, 1961). Whether it is a central component is questioned for the same reason that health was questioned; i.e., it, too, is included in the theoretical definition of need. The concept as presented by Orlando is in part operationally defined since improvement can be based on what the general state of the individual was when the nursing process started.

Improvement can be considered a central component, because if it does not exist, nursing is either inadequate, ineffective or nonexistent. Improvement, like health, is an important part of the measured outcome of nursing action and is not governed by patient prognosis. Improvement is also important to Orlando because of her interest in quality of nursing care. Improvement of care has been a major impetus for her work. Improvement is not only the end result but also the initial goal—*"whatever principles are brought to bear on the nursing situation, the ultimate aim is to bring about improvement in the nursing care of patients"* (Orlando, p 8, 1961).

Nursing is the most important central component of the model. This concept is directly related to each of the others and the relationship is described in the discussion of each of the other components. Nursing is explicated in an earlier section as one of the basic concepts.

Types of Concepts

According to Hardy (1974), Orlando's concept of patient and need are nonvariable because they are clearly defined; i.e., someone is either a patient or not, there is either a need or no need. Nursing, health, and interaction are largely invariable because they exist or they do not exist. They possess characteristics of being variable because they do change and vary but primarily because of their relationships with improvement and validation. These latter two concepts are considered nonvariable because once again they are either present or absent. Even though improvement involves various dimensions, these are not important in the propositions posed by Orlando's model.

A similar distinction can be made using Dubin's (1978) discussion. Although some of Orlando's concepts have elements of being variable, they are considered attributes, i.e., distinguished by the quality of being present. Dubin emphasizes that with the use of variable units, attention is focused on one possible combination of relationships between two variables. By using all attribute concepts, Orlando avoids this. However, there are still major restrictions since in some cases empirical data related to three of the four possible combinations would have no relevance for her theory; e.g., a patient with a need would require nursing, but a patient without a need, a non-patient without a need, and a non-patient with a need would not require nursing care. At the same time, testing of such possible combinations could be a means of identifying other areas of concern to nurses. The numerous combinations would definitely have an effect on the structure of Orlando's model, the kinds of predictions generated, and the extensiveness of the tests that can be made of it.

Orlando's concepts are distinguished as real concepts as opposed to nominal ones because they either have or it is possible for them to have empirical indicators. The advantage is that the parts of her theory should be able to be tested; the disadvantages lie in the lack of scientific imaginative extension, i.e., there is no potential for identification of the realms of the unknown (Dubin, 1978).

Nursing is considered a collective concept and the other central concepts discussed are member concepts of that collective. Dubin (1978) says that the purpose of making this distinction is to designate many things showing at least one common characteristic and to be able to treat them as a unit (concept) in a theory.

Orlando's concepts are considered associative units. According to Dubin, this is a property characteristic of a thing in only some of its conditions; there is an absent value. If there were an absent value for any of the concepts, however, nursing would not exist.

Relationships of Concepts

The relationships between concepts have been discussed with each concept. However, examination of all of the relationships would allow for the logical adequacy of the theory to be assessed. Use of Hardy's (1974) types of relationships indicates that many of the relationships are necessary or conditional. Examples are: when there is a patient, and only when there is a patient, can there be nursing. A patient must have a need for there to be nursing (conditional). If there is nursing interaction, the needs of the patient are met (necessary).

Logical Adequacy

The sign of the relationships, whether there is a positive or inverse relationship, allows for further examination of the logical deduction of the relationships. The evaluation of a theory's structure is facilitated when the concepts and relationship between concepts are formalized (Hardy, 1974). Although this is not always true for Orlando's model, logical adequacy can still be assessed to some degree. Actually Orlando's theory is very logical. The missing steps in logic can be supplied with consideration of her theoretical and operational definitions. When a patient has a need, a nurse interacts validating both the need and the help provided. As a direct result, there is an improvement in health. If any part does not exist, then there really is no nursing because a lack of or inadequate type of nursing is the same as no nursing. The implied internal relationships are logical but as Hardy (1974) says, a relationship which is true according to logic is not necessarily true empirically. Further reformulation and refinement of internal relationship, not necessarily by the author, would be beneficial.

There is consistency throughout the theory. There were several points that might be questioned initially. When Orlando speaks of person as a behaving human organism with the end result of physical and mental health, there appears to be a lack of socialness. A behaving human demands a social element by its very nature and certainly this element has great influence over a sense of adequacy and well being. Orlando also attributes much importance to interaction, a social behavior. Although there is consistency, the empirical adequacy may be questioned on certain social points, e.g., family centered care.

In current nursing practice there may be a certain amount of unacceptability when it comes to the physician having total responsibility for a patient's care. This is an interpretation by Orlando; of course, interpretation can be adapted to the time. However, even here Orlando is consistent. When she speaks of the nursing task of using medically prescribed activities, she is using them for the patient and not carrying out orders for the physician. According to Orlando, this is logical because if the patient were able to carry out the diagnostic treatment plan alone, in all probability the nurse would not become involved in the first place. The resulting inference seems to be an area where Orlando may have an inconsistent perspective. There could be distinct areas of involvement for the nurse in the above case, e.g., teaching, explaining, preparing, etc. A related question arises in terms of how Orlando distinguishes medicine and nursing. She stresses the importance of the patient's capacity to use the treatment and preventive measures and that this is the responsibility of the nurse. The inconsistency appears mainly because this might well be interpreted as prevention on the part of the nurse when prevention is the realm of the physician, according to Orlando. She also speaks of nurses explaining, informing, directing, instructing, etc., in their practice. These activities take on a different perspective than her concept of interaction. Unfortunately her emphasis on interaction tends to hide the fact that she does recognize other aspects of nursing practice.

The scope of Orlando's model is limited. She does deal with concepts which in and of themselves represent a broad scope, but by her definition she narrows the scope and thus the potential significance for nursing. Orlando's model does cover both biological and behavioral observations and also has potential for explaining their relationship. Unfortunately, Orlando emphasized verbal interaction so much that the other parts of her theory are underdeveloped, particularly in the area of biological observations. Ellis (1968) states that for nursing, the scope should be judged in terms of that which is pertinent and the circumstances which cause an individual to be labeled by the concept patient. Since Orlando simply says that the patient is a person under medical treatment or supervision, indications are that the scope is narrow.

Orlando's model does have some complexity. Directly and indirectly she deals with a number of variables and a number of relationships which give a theory complexity (Ellis, 1968). Although implicit and explicit postulations appear simple and readily apparent, they are not always so. The idea and value of patient validation seem very obvious but validation often does not occur or is not recognized in clinical practice as being that important. When validation is used, it can and has stimulated new insights.

One of the most valuable characteristics of Orlando's model is that it is useful for developing and guiding clinical practice. This value has been discussed by Ellis (1968). The most clinically useful aspects are patient validation and verbal interaction. These nursing practices have been demonstrated as very valuable in the course of effective nursing care.

Orlando's model is also capable of generating new information because a number of hypotheses can be derived and there is a potential for discovery of new information, and verification and stimulation of new ways of viewing old problems. Ellis (1968) says that theory is significant for nursing if it can enlighten nursing practice. Orlando's model on this basis alone is considered significant.

EXTERNAL ANALYSIS OF THE MODEL

Nursing Research

Orlando's model has been developed from studying experiences in nursing and teaching. Orlando identified a goal of nursing as the development of knowledge which is distinctly nursing. She views the systematic study of nursing situations as necessary to formulate principles which when applied to the nursing process can be effective in helping patients, and which give strong potential for research. Understanding how practices help or do not help the patient is how the nurse develops and improves her knowledge and skill in practice. Orlando sees the study of how the nurse affects the patient and how this influences the course of the patient's condition as exciting and promising in the further development of nursing research.

Orlando says that the most promising area in the development of nursing research is how the nurse affects the patient and how this influences the course of the patient's condition. Subsequently, in the early 1960s, after Orlando's book was published, a number of studies attempted to accomplish this. Anderson, Mertz and Leonard (1965) looked at the patient-centered nursing approach and its beneficial effect on the patient's welfare during the admission process. Similarly, Orlando's deliberative nursing process to ascertain and meet the patient's immediate needs was studied by: Bochnak (1963) in relation to relief of pain; Dumas and Leonard (1963) in relation to post-operative vomiting; Dye (1963) in relation to patient's immediate need for help; Fischelis (1963) in relation to labels placed on patient's behaviors; and, Rhymes (1964), Tryon and Leonard (1964), and Tryon (1963) in relation to interaction between the nurse and patient. Cameron (1963) explored the nurse-patient interaction and Faulkner (1963) looked at communication of need. Elder (1963) and Gowan and Morris (1964) both found that many patients are unable to communicate their needs but that effective nursing interaction remedied this.

Unless there is some awareness of the practicality of viewing the relation of professional purpose to the mode of theorizing, the development of theory could constitute just one more academic distraction for nursing (Dickoff & James, 1968). However, as was just described, Orlando does advocate research in nursing practice, causing theory to be not only useful, but also to stimulate the generation of new insights and new ideas.

Nursing Practice

Models of nursing practice can be derived from research upon scientifically supported generalizations relative to practice. Nursing principles derived from the model relate to the unique context of nursing. Whether a nursing model is significant concerns its usefulness for practice (Ellis, 1968). The concepts and propositions in Orlando's model offer clear and relevant guides to practice.

Throughout the text Orlando consistently focuses on the purpose of nursing as she defines it—nursing data are examined, discussed and directed toward the identification of nursing function, process, and principles of professional nursing practice. In each contact the nurse repeats a process of learning how to help the individual patient. The nurse's own individuality and that of the patient require that the nurse go through this each time the nurse gives nursing care. In order for the nurse to develop and maintain the professional character of nursing practice, the nurse must know and be able to validate how actions help or do not help the patient. In this process, the nurse also validates that the patient does or does not require the nurse's help at a given time.

Orlando supplies numerous practice examples; one of her clinical examples is described here: a mother is instructed to hold her newborn infant "close" and not between her knees as she was doing. Ensuing episodes of anoxemia are noted on the day after the nurse's suggestion. The nurse observes the mother's handling of the infant and finds that the mother is holding the infant in a "tourniquet-like" hold. The nurse discusses with the mother her usual way of holding an infant and finds it adequate. The mother and nurse then discuss that the mother's prior method of holding the baby will alleviate the problem.

The understanding required by the nurse before she could help the mother was distinct from the understanding which would explain her observations and activity. The principles that blueness means oxygen depletion, that babies need tender loving care, and that the unconscious may be manifest in observed behavior, while valid in themselves, were not sufficient or even appropriate to the unique and immediate experience of the patient and the nurse. What happened between them, how it happened, and its relationship to the process of helping the patient was the understanding which was needed.

The principles relative to the depletion and restoration of oxygen and the emotional health of infants were the first which were applied in the situation with the mother. The nurse, preoccupied with the prior instruction, was prevented from finding out what was happening to the patient. It was almost as if these principles conditioned the nurse's first thoughts when she observed the patient. Since the principles were valid, the nurse did not find it necessary to question or hesitate in applying them. Few nurses would question that babies should be held close, that blue coloring beneath the surface of the skin means oxygen depletion, or that the mother at some level rejected her child (Orlando, p 2-3, 1961).

Jacox (1974) discusses some important factors in the development of nursing practice theory. Theory must fit the nursing empirical reality; Orlando's was developed from this. There is a necessity to generalize about situations. Orlando's are generalizations; they cover diverse practice situations. Theory should be couched in terms which can be readily understood by practitioners; Orlando's terms are understandable. Theory should include specific guidelines for control in the practice setting; using Orlando's theory, the practitioner can control situations.

Nursing Education

The purpose of the *Dynamic Nurse-Patient Relationship* was to offer the student of professional nursing a theory of effective nursing practice. Orlando's book was the product of a four-year grant which identified the content of instruction, the teaching process, and the learning environment needed by students for the development of a professional nursing role. The teaching process and learning environment needed by nursing students was not discussed in this book. The elements of a nursing model provide guidance in process of curriculum development and also unify and coordinate all aspects of the program (Riehl & Roy, 1974). Many of the content areas that would be dictated are included in curricula designed after other theories, e.g., interaction, recognition and identification of needs, patient validation. Nursing content for instruction of students provides a foundation for education of a dynamic nurse.

SUMMARY

Orlando's model, although not developed to the extent of the later models, does offer a guide for nursing practice. One of the most valuable aspects of the model has been the critical element of patient validation of what needs exist and whether the nurse's actions are successful in helping meet these needs.

Orlando's concept of patient involves those persons under medical treatment or supervision. Nurses are professionally concerned only with those patients who have needs which they cannot meet comfortably on their own. The nurse's goal is the improvement of the patient's mental and physical health or comfort, with a sense of adequacy and well-being. This goal is achieved when the nurse supplies the help patients require in order for their needs to be met. Intersubjectivity is questioned in regard to the concept of patient based on current empirical reality. The concept of interaction is heavily emphasized by Orlando, to the extent that other important aspects of the model are overlooked.

Orlando's model is logically adequate and consistent and, although the scope of her model is narrow, there is complexity and the usefulness is significant. Orlando views the study of how the nurse affects the patient and how this influences the course of the patient's condition as promising in nursing research. Thus, in conclusion, the concepts and principles in Orlando's model offer clear and relevant guides to nursing practice. The purpose of *The Dynamic Nurse-Patient Relationship* was to offer the professional nursing student a model for effective nursing practice; this seems to have been achieved.

REFERENCES

Anderson BJ, Mertz H, Leonard RC: Two experimental tests of a patient-centered admission process. Nursing Research, Vol 14, pp 151-157, 1965

Bochnak MA: The effect of an automatic and deliberative process of nursing activity, on the relief of patients' pain: A clinical experiment. Nursing Research, Vol 12, pp 191-192, 1963

Cameron J: An exploratory study of the verbal responses of the nurse patient interactions. Nursing Research, Vol 12, p 192, 1963

Dickoff J, James P: A theory of theories: A position paper. Nursing Research, Vol 17, pp 197-203, 1968

Dumas RG, Leonard RC: The effects of nursing on the incidence of post-operative vomiting. Nursing Research, Vol 12, pp 12-15, 1963

Dye MD: A descriptive study of conditions conducive to an effective process of nursing activity. Nursing Research, Vol 12, p 194, 1963

Elder RG: What is the patient saying? Nursing Forum, Vol 2, pp 25-37, 1963

Ellis R: Characteristics of significant theories. Nursing Research, Vol 17, No 3, pp 217-222, 1968

Faulkner SA: A descriptive study of needs communicated to the nurse by some mothers on a post-partum service. Nursing Research, Vol 12, p 260, 1963

Fischelis MC: An exploratory study of labels nurses attach to patient behavior and their effect on nursing activities. Nursing Research, Vol 13, p 195, 1963

Gowan NI, Morris M: Nurses responses to expressed patients' needs. Nursing Research, Vol 13, pp 68-71, 1964

Hardy M: Theories: Components, development, evaluation. Nursing Research, Vol 23, pp 100-107, 1974

Jacox A: Theory construction in nursing: An overview. Nursing Research, Vol 23, pp 4-13, 1974

Kuhn T: The Structure of Scientific Revolutions. The University of Chicago Press, Chicago, Illinois, 1970

Orlando IJ: The Dynamic Nurse-Patient Relationship. G.P. Putnam's Sons, New York, 1961

Orlando IJ: The Discipline and Teaching of Nursing Process. G.P. Putnam's Sons, New York, 1972

Pelletier IO: The patient's predicament and nursing function. Psychiatric Opinion, Vol 4, pp 25-30, 1967

Reynolds PD: A Primer in Theory Construction. The Bobbs-Merrill Co., Inc., New York, 1971

Rhymes J: A description of nurse-patient interaction in effective nursing activity. Nursing Research, Vol 13, No 4, 1964

Riehl JP, Roy C: Conceptual Models for Nursing Practice. Appleton-Century-Crofts, New York, 1974

Tryon PA: An experiment of the effect of patients participation in planning the administration of a nursing procedure. Nursing Research, Vol 12, pp 262-265, 1963

Tryon PA, Leonard RC: An experiment of the effect of patients participation on the outcome of a nursing procedure. Nursing Forum, Vol 3, pp 79-89, 1964

5

WIEDENBACH'S MODEL

Edith Raleigh

INTRODUCTION

Wiedenbach's model grew out of forty years of experience in nursing, mostly maternity nursing. As a result of her own experiences, she began asking questions about the nature and practice of nursing. Her experiences as a teacher made the quest to find answers to her questions about nursing more imperative. Her position at Yale University enabled her to have frequent dialogues with others involved in theory development such as Orlando, Dickoff, and James. In this environment her ideas solidified into the model she presents in her book, *Clinical Nursing: A Helping Art* (Wiedenbach, 1964). It is interesting to note that the women's movement, which has brought greater opportunities for men as well as women, had not yet had an influence upon nursing, or Wiedenbach's thinking, as evidenced by the following statement:

> "People may differ in their concept of nursing, but few would disagree that nursing is nurturing or caring for someone in a *motherly* fashion" (Wiedenbach, 1964, p 1, emphasis added).

An initial question considered here is, can this work be classified as a theory of nursing science and practice? According

to Ellis (1968), a theory may be defined as "a coherent set of hypothetical, conceptual, and pragmatic principles forming a general
frame of reference for a field of inquiry" (p 217). Hardy (p 104,
1974) defines a conceptual model as "a simplified representation
of a theory or of certain complex events, structure, or systems."
Wiedenbach's model will be examined in light of guidelines for
analysis and evaluation of theory and will be found to better fit
the definition of a model. In this analysis and evaluation, it is
important to keep in mind that Wiedenbach's model is one of
the earlier nursing models. Therefore, it is not nor is it expected
to be as fully developed as later nursing models.

BASIC CONSIDERATIONS

The analysis of Wiedenbach's model will begin with an
examination of the basic concepts of person, health and nursing
that have come to be identified with the science of nursing. It is
important that concepts within a theoretical statement be defined precisely. Once concepts are defined, their meanings are
understood, however, only within the framework of the theory
of which they are a part (Hardy, 1973). With these guidelines in
mind, the concepts basic to Wiedenbach's model of nursing will
be examined.

Definition of Nursing, Person, Health

Wiedenbach (1964) defines nursing as "a helping art." It
is a "deliberate blend of thoughts, feelings, and overt actions ...
practiced in relation to an individual who is in need of help"
(p 11). The area of responsibility that is unique to the nurse is that
of focusing on the patient's perception of his or her condition.
Nursing is patient-centered, designed to assist the patient when
the individual perceives a need for assistance. The activity of
nursing is triggered by a behavioral stimulus from the individual.
Wiedenbach has identified in part the domain of nursing by
defining it as the "now" or the actual moment when the nurse is
in contact with the patient.

Wiedenbach defines person, or man, as a functioning being.
She states that the ability to cope is something that is inherent in
the human being. Health is not defined specifically in Wiedenbach's model.

Description of Nursing Activity

According to Wiedenbach there are four elements in clinical nursing: 1) philosophy, 2) purpose, 3) practice, and 4) art. She states that nursing is rooted in an explicit philosophy. She describes three points that are basic to this philosophy of nursing.

1. Reverence for the gift of life.
2. Respect for the dignity, worth, autonomy, and individuality of each human being.
3. Resolution to act dynamically in relation to one's beliefs (p 16).

Clinical nursing is directed toward fulfillment of a specific purpose. That purpose is to assist the individual to surmount the obstacles which impede competent response to the requirements of his/her condition, environment, and/or situation. The element of purpose can be stated more succinctly: nursing's goal is "to meet the need (that) the individual is experiencing as a need-for-help" (Wiedenbach, p 15, 1964). Thus, the focus of the nurse is the patient's immediate perceptions as well as physical needs.

The third element, practice, is defined as "overt action, directed by disciplined thoughts and feelings toward meeting the patient's need-for-help" (Wiedenbach, p 23, 1964). It is supported by nursing administration, nursing education, and nursing organizations. Clinical practice is carried on within limits that are both general and unique. The nurse focuses on and acts as a result of the patient's behavior which is a response to his/her perception of the situation. Wiedenbach describes the practice of clinical nursing as patient-centered as well as goal directed and involving deliberate action.

There are three integral components to the practice of clinical nursing. Knowledge encompasses everything that has been comprehended. Judgment involves the ability of the nurse to make sound decisions. Skills represents "the nurse's ability to achieve the appropriate outcomes."

Wiedenbach describes four phases to the practice of clinical nursing: 1) identification of the patient's experienced need-for-help, 2) ministration of the help that is needed, 3) validation that the help provided was indeed the help needed, and 4) coordination of the resources for help and of the help provided. Coordination involves reporting, consulting, and conferring.

The fourth element of clinical nursing is art. This is defined by Wiedenbach (1964) as the "application of knowledge and skill toward meeting a need-for-help experienced by a patient" (p 36). When the nurse is in contact with the patient, the purpose of the nurse determines the nurse's role as helper. Whether the nurse's process turns out to be a helping one depends on how clearly she/he perceives the purpose, on the deliberate applicaton of the purpose to actions, and on the exercise of judgment in applying the principles of helping to the actions. In this way, the art of nursing is comprised of deliberative action which is triggered by the patient's behavior. The deliberative action is "based on the nurse's perceptions and feelings but is tempered by the exercise of judgment in applying principles of helping in light of the nurse's overall purpose with respect to her patient" (Wiedenbach, p 42, 1964).

This concept of nursing is very detailed with elements, components, and phases of components. It does, however, meet the requirement identified by Ellis (1968) for a significant nursing theory in that "nursing is not defined by the activities of the nurse but by what the patient receives from them" (p 218). In Wiedenbach's model, nursing is defined as nursing actions which aid the individual in overcoming obstacles which interfere with his/her ability to respond independently. Wiedenbach's nursing is patient-centered.

Understanding of Person

The person, in Wiedenbach's model, is a "physically-physiologically-psychologically" reacting being whose responses may be self-willed or involuntary. The attention given to the understanding of person is limited. It is clear that the focus of nursing is the patient, that is an individual who is receiving some kind of help from a health-field professional.

The individual is seen as competent and (generally) able to determine if a need for help is being experienced. Nurses need to intervene only when there is an obstacle which prevents the individual from satisfactorily coping with the demands being placed upon him or her by the situation.

One may deduce from these statements that Wiedenbach views person as a unified whole and that obstacles in one area influence the quality of coping of the entire individual. It is important for a significant nursing theory to define person in this way since it is characteristic of nursing in contrast to all other disciplines (Johnson, 1968).

Understanding of Health

The concept of health is not specifically addressed in Wiedenbach's model. The object of nursing actions is the patient which, according to Wiedenbach's definition, implies a health-related concern. Aside from this basic understanding, the concept of health is not discussed or defined. It seems to be assumed that the definition of health in relation to nursing is well-understood. This is problematic in the development of this model because it is important for clarity and applicability to define concepts (Jacox, 1974). Since health is considered a concept which is basic to nursing theory, a clearer definition is needed.

Relationships Among Concepts of Person, Environment, Health, and Nursing

Wiedenbach does not directly define the concept of environment. A definiton can however be inferred from her discussion of professional nursing activity; in this discussion the concepts of person and nursing have major significance for the model. Nursing exists to meet the human need-for-help. Without this cue to action there would be no nursing. Wiedenbach does not go so far, however, as to say that the human need-for-help could not be met without nursing. It would seem logical that nursing, as she defines it, focuses on and exists for meeting this need. If there were not a discipline designed to meet that need, then it could conceivably go unmet.

Description of the Basic Concepts

Wiedenbach concentrates the development of her model on the concept of nursing. With the exception of the need-for-help, the basic components of the model are derived from professional nursing practice. The need-for-help as experienced by the patient is the stimulus for nursing activity. The professional nursing activity that results is in the form of nursing practice and nursing art. Nursing practice is the activity in which the nurse engages in response to the patient's need-for-help. Nursing art is an analysis of information that is based on the nurse's perceptions and professional judgment. The principles of helping are three points which are said to be characteristic of helping behavior. These basic components are discussed in greater detail below.

Relationships of Basic Concepts to Person, Environment, Health, and Nursing

In Wiedenbach's model there is obvious interplay between clinical nursing (and its many components) and the basic concept of person. Nursing exists for the purpose of meeting the need-for-help as experienced by person. Person, a normally functioning, capable being, calls upon nursing when obstacles interfere with the ability to cope and a need-for-help is experienced. The practice, art, and philosophy of clinical nursing are the means by which the nurse intervenes to meet the need-for-help.

The environment comes into play in this model only when it may contain or produce an obstacle resulting in a need-for-help. On the other hand, environment may contain or produce the elements necessary for nursing ministration to the need-for-help. The concept of health does not interrelate with the Wiedenbach components. It is not clear that the need-for-help is health-related. The more recent emphasis in nursing models, that health represents more than the absence of disease, is not as evident in the model. This conceptualization however which "permits health to be thought of as a dynamic state or process ... rather than a static either/or entity" (Carper, p 15, 1978) would be suited to Wiedenbach's conceptualization of nursing. This definition of health would articulate very well with her concept of the focus of nursing as being the patient's perceptions. If the patient perceives a health-related problem, then the nurse would treat it as such.

INTERNAL THEORY ANALYSIS

A theory is generally defined as a systematically related set of statements, including some law-like generalizations, that is empirically testable (Rudner, 1966). To determine if an espoused theory meets these criteria, it is necessary to analyze the relationships among the components. Since a theory may be differentiated from other forms of knowledge by 1) the nature of the terms used, and 2) the character of its internal relations (Walker, 1971), attention is now turned to the internal consistency of the model. This internal analysis will involve an examination of the various components of Wiedenbach's model and the manner in which these components are interrelated.

Underlying Assumptions

Assumptions are relational statements that ordinarily are not subjected to empirical testing (Dickoff and James, 1968b). Wiedenbach identifies four assumptions about person:

1. Each human being is endowed with unique potential to develop—within himself—resources which enable him to maintain and sustain himself.
2. The human being basically strives toward self-direction and relative independence and desires not only to make best use of his capabilities and potentialities but to fulfill his responsibilities.
3. Self-awareness and self-acceptance are essential to the individual's sense of integrity and self-worth.
4. Whatever the individual does represents his best judgment at the moment of his doing it (p 17).

Other assumptions in the model are implicit. Wiedenbach assumes that nurses ascribe to what she calls a philosophy of nursing. Although it may be true that nurses base their practice on a similar underlying philosophy, whether or not it is the one she presents is not known. Wiedenbach's statement of philosophy is seen by Walker (1971) as a statement of her personal beliefs and attitudes toward (her) profession. It is important to note, however, that goals in patient care are not value-free, and these values may be reflected in the kinds of theory developed (Jacox, 1974). Also, according to Ellis (1968), it is necessary to recognize and make explicit the values implied in the theory. This is what Wiedenbach has done. Assumptions inherent in the principle of inconsistency-consistency (to be discussed below) are that life is an orderly process and that the human being is geared to orderly living. Although these conditions have not been identified by Wiedenbach as assumptions, they clearly fall into that category.

Central Components of the Model

An examination of the major components of a model is a critical part of its analysis. According to Hardy (1978), evaluation involves considering its logical and empirical adequacy and its

usefulness and significance. In order to do this the interrelationships of the components must be assessed. These components should have operational definitions if the theory is to
be empirically testable (Fawcett, 1978). With these guidelines in
mind, the major components of Wiedenbach's model (need-for-
help, nursing practice, nursing art, and principles of helping)
are discussed.

Definitions of These Components

Need-For-Help

The identification by the professional nurse of a need-for-
help experienced by the patient is the focus of nursing. This need-
for-help must be recognized or perceived by the patient before
nursing can begin. This is an essential component of the theory
since nursing exists for the purpose of helping the individual.
Also, this concept relates to the nurse's area of responsibility in
that the identification of the need-for-help must come from the
patient's experience. The patient must perceive the need-for-help
before the nurse can intervene. The need-for-help can be operationally defined as follows: Any need identified by the patient as
one that may be met by requesting (verbally or non-verbally) help
from a nurse. This concept, need-for-help, is a relational unit by
Dubin's (1978) definition since its value can be determined only
in relation to other properties such as competence and independence.

Nursing Practice

This concept gives a name to that activity which results from
a need-for-help as perceived by the patient and the nurse. The
practice of nursing is directed toward meeting the patient's need-
for-help. Factors that influence the practice of nursing are the
nurse's knowledge, judgment, and skills. In addition, the purpose
and philosophy of nursing provide the framework for the practice
of nursing. The components of practice or the specific activities
in which the nurse engages during the practice of nursing are
1) identification of the need-for-help, 2) ministration of the help
needed, 3) coordination of resources, and 4) validation that the
help provided was the help needed. Nursing practice is also a relational unit (Dubin, 1978) since it has no value or property outside of the need-for-help experienced by the patient.

Nursing Art

The concept of the art of nursing is defined by Wiedenbach as the use of knowledge and skill for the purpose of achieving the desired outcome. In an attempt to further clarify the concept, Wiedenbach states that it is comprised of deliberative action which seems to be action based on intuition. This is a professional intuition which is influenced by knowledge and judgment. She states that prior to deliberative action the nurse analyzes information based on perceptions, and feelings, and the exercise of judgment while keeping in mind the overall purpose with respect to the patient.

Art is a recognized part of nursing. Abdellah (1969) states that the art of nursing "concerns itself with intuitive and technical skills . . . and also the more important supportive aspects of nursing" (p 69). Carper (1978) calls it the "esthetic pattern of knowing" (p 16). The concept of art and esthetic meaning requires a "fluid and open approach" making "possible a wider consideration of conditions, situations, and experiences in nursing that may properly be called esthetic, including the creative process of discovery in the empirical pattern of knowing" (p 16). It would seem, therefore, that the art of nursing is defined by the results of the esthetic knowledge. The actions taken by the nurse to meet the patient's need-for-help give meaning and substance to the art of nursing. Carper (1978) states that for "the action taken (by the nurse) to have an esthetic quality," there must be an "active transformation of . . . the patient's behavior into a direct . . . perception of what is significant in it—that is, what need is being expressed by the behavior" (p 17). The art of nursing and nursing practice cannot be separated. The art of nursing is evident only through the practice of nursing; they are interwoven. As such, nursing art is a relational unit (Dubin, 1978) since it has no property outside of nursing practice. The art of nursing cannot exist without nursing activity and patient need-for-help.

Principles Of Helping

Wiedenbach identifies the following three characteristics of helping which she calls principles. These are: 1) principle of inconsistency-consistency; 2) principle of purposeful perseverance; and, 3) principle of self-extension. The principle of inconsistency-consistency implies that based on knowledge and prior experience, one has a concept of "normal" or "expected" occurrences. When behavior or circumstances vary from the expected, one is aware of an inconsistency that acts as a stimulus to warn that something is out of order. This is also a relational unit; consistency cannot be defined without inconsistency and vice versa.

The principle of purposeful perseverance suggests that the nurse will persevere to identify a patient's need-for-help when one is suspected. This principle involves a number of skills and commitments which are fundamental to the nurse, such as a genuine desire to help, judgment, and resourcefulness in communicating and intervening therapeutically. Perseverance is an associative unit since it may have a zero value, that is, giving up, and may range from perseverance for a short time to perseverance to death.

The third principle, self-extension, involves using resources outside of oneself for help, guidance, or advice. This principle also involves the inclusion of the patient in the planning and caring. Self-extension is also an associative unit since one may elect not to self-extend or any degree in between.

Relative Importance of the Components

Need-for-help, nursing practice and nursing art carry equal weight in their importance to the model. These three components are interrelated and have no meaning aside from their interaction. The principles of helping are not so important to the model. They add depth and expression to nursing practice and art but play a minor role in the flow of professional nursing activity.

Relationships Among Components

The term "principle" has been used very loosely in nursing literature. What is frequently meant by a "principle" is a "proposition." The definition of a proposition is a statement of a constant relationship between two or more concepts or between two or more facts. In addition, propositions that state causal relationships are called axioms. When the explanations of Wiedenbach's principles are examined, one can identify that they do, in fact, state a constant, relationship between two or more concepts. The first principle states a relationship among expected occurrences, variance from the expected, and inconsistency. It is clearly causal in its relationships. Variance from the expected causes the nurse to interpret an inconsistency or disorder in the occurrence. The second principle relates perseverance and a need-for-help. The third principle relates the nurse to resourcefulness. These principles of helping fit into the model in that they temper the nurse's perceptions and feelings which precede deliberative action. Figure 5.1 is a diagrammatic representative of Wiedenbach's model in an attempt to clarify the relationships of the concepts included in the model.

Analysis of Consistency

Wiedenbach's model is internally consistent. Those concepts that are defined have clear definitions. In addition, the assumptions are consistent with the concepts. For example, her assumptions about person are consistent with her definition of person. The relationships between the concepts are also consistent.

Hardy (1978) suggests diagramming the concepts to clarify the linkages and to identify gaps and contradictions. Figure 5.1 demonstrates that the major components can be linked and that directionality can be assigned. The connections between the obstacles for the patient and the nurse's paths of interpretation are somewhat difficult to diagram, which leads to the conclusion that this is a model, not yet a theory.

Analysis of Adequacy

Hardy (1974) identifies specific types of adequacy for which theories should be evaluated. The validity of the assumptions and meaning of the concepts as well as operational and empirical adequacy should be addressed. Specifically, the extent to which there are operational definitions for the concepts which would permit measurement and the extent to which these definitions accurately reflect the theoretical concepts can be evaluated.

The assumptions made by Wiedenbach would be generally accepted as true with the exception of the assumption that all nurses adhere to a similar philosophy. In this day of evolving ideas regarding quality of life, similar philosophical positions may not be generally accepted. The concepts of nursing practice, consistency-inconsistency, and self-extension are operationally defined so as to permit measurement and to accurately reflect the theoretical concept. The concepts of nursing art and purposeful perseverance are not operationally defined although there is an attempt made to do so. The concept need-for-help is operationally defined in such a way that it accurately reflects the theoretical concept; however, the definition may not apply to all instances.

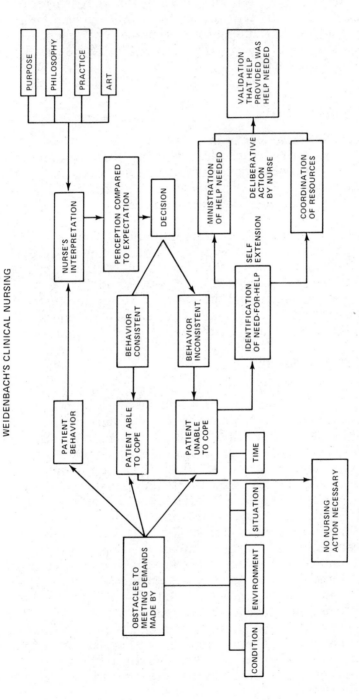

Figure 5.1. This diagram portrays the interrelationships of the concepts in Wiedenbach's model. Obstacles result in patient behavior which is characteristic of coping or non-coping. The patient's behavior acts as a stimulus to professional nursing practice resulting in an interpretation of the behavior as coping or non-coping. Coping behavior requires no nursing activity. Non-coping behavior leads to identification of the need-for-help and deliberative action by the nurse.

When a nurse suspects a need-for-help, this must be confirmed by the patient that such a need exists. It can be recalled that the need-for-help must exist from the patient's perspective. This may be difficult to validate in the infant or comatose patient.

Duffey and Muhlenkamp (1974) suggest that in analyzing a theory one should pose the question "what is the origin of the problem?" (p 573). Wiedenbach's model deals with a need-for-help originating from obstacles which prevent the individual from meeting his/her own needs. In keeping with this concrete conceptualization, the problems originate from empirical observation. This appears to be the result of inductive theory development. Wiedenbach began with her practice experiences and developed and interrelated concepts from an analysis of that clinical experience.

Another criterion for assessing a theory is that it "fulfills the purpose for which the theory was proposed . . . as the purpose of the theory varies, the structure or level of the theory varies" (Dickoff and James, p 198, 1968b). Wiedenbach's model was proposed to describe professional nursing practice. It came out of her observations of what it is that nurses do. It fulfills the purpose for which it was proposed; that is, description of professional nursing practice. In this role it may approach theory at the second level; that is, factor-relating or situation-depicting theory. The model relates the various concepts that Wiedenbach identified as components of professional nursing practice. It does not predict the situations and, thus, could not be considered third level theory which is situation-relating or predictive theory.

A criterion that Blalock (1969) uses for theory evaluation is that it must combine features of being sufficiently general and complex, explicitly formulated. Jacox (1974) adds that "for a theory to be 'sufficiently general and complex,' it should fall somewhere between explaining a very small part of the empirical world and trying to explain everything about a particular science or discipline with a single theory" (p 11). With Jacox's clarification in mind, Wiedenbach's model does fall somewhere in the middle range. It is not all-inclusive. It does not attempt to predict or produce situations in nursing practice, only to explain the situations that take place.

By Ellis' (1968) criteria, Wiedenbach's model does have scope. It covers a number of concepts, both physical and psychological. The need-for-help may come from either realm. Another criterion Ellis identifies is complexity. Wiedenbach's model does have a certain degree of complexity in that it relates some very complex phenomena which are characteristics of professional nursing practice. The last two criteria for evaluating a theory, according to Ellis, are usefulness and ability to generate new information. Wiedenbach's model is useful in that it describes and explains the activities and interactions known as professional nursing practice. In this sense it is heuristic in that it generates new information by raising questions about Wiedenbach's postulations.

EXTERNAL THEORY ANALYSIS

Empirical relevance is an important criterion for evaluating a theory. One needs to consider how the theory fits into the real world; it must lend itself to empirical testing. External theory analysis requires consideration of the type of research, education, and practice indicated by the theory.

Relationship to Nursing Research

A theory must be testable to be judged as valid. To determine how accurately the propositions fit empirical reality, the theory must be tested in the empirical world (Jacox, 1974). A good theory can be the framework for a productive exploration of phenomena and testing of hypotheses. It can indicate areas that would be more likely to result in significant gains in knowledge (Abdellah, 1969). In addition, a theory should generate new information and hypotheses. Even if the hypotheses are difficult to test, the theory can add to current understanding of phenomena (Ellis, 1968).

Research should be done in the context of a theory if its addition to the body of knowledge is to be meaningful. Similarly, the impact that the research may have on the theory should be clearly understood (Dickoff and James, 1968a). It is the conceptual framework inherent in a theory that dictates the type of research design which is appropriate (Batey, 1971). Research in which nurses participated, prior to Wiedenbach's formulation of clinical nursing, focused on medical problems. Their efforts tended to be aimed at assisting the individual to adjust to the diagnostic and therapeutic techniques under study. Wiedenbach's model of nursing identifies the focus of nursing research which should be the patient's response to the health care experience. The conceptual framework for clinical nursing clearly points to the nurse's concern being facilitation of the patient's efforts to respond capably to the demands made upon him or her by his/her condition, environment, situation, and time.

Wiedenbach suggests that studies that would be consistent with this framework of nursing would focus on promoting family relationships, controlling elements associated with disabling conditions, and facilitating sensible health practices. Studies that are within the nurse's area of responsibility are those that explore the nurse's responses to patients and the patient's responses to them. Additionally, nursing research focuses on clarifying concepts related to the patients' perceptions of their circumstances including their needs-for-help, identifying factors in nursing practice that can be useful in producing beneficial outcomes in patients and for meeting their needs-for-help, and developing instruments which measure the capacity and well-being of the patient.

Relationship to Nursing Education

Wiedenbach's model is based upon a broad understanding of person and society. Application of the model requires knowledge of the "normal" and the "abnormal," a thorough understanding of human psychology, and competence in procedural and communication skills. Additionally, the practitioner must have developed sound judgment for making decisions regarding interpretation of human behavior and implementation of interventions. This prescribes a general education for nursing's professional practitioners. Graduate education would focus on developing greater skills in the nursing process; that is, identification, ministration, and validation. Wiedenbach writes of nursing education as a service for nursing practice, a separate entity, and does not clearly relate them as interdependent. Nursing education is much more than a service to practice. The type and quality of a nurse's practice finds its origin in the type and quality of that nurse's education.

Relationship to Professional Nursing Practice

Glaser and Strauss (1967) identify four requirements for practice theory. It must:

1. Closely relate and apply to the daily realities of the area in which it is to be used.
2. Be understandable to the people using it.

3. Be general enough to cover the ever-changing practice situations, yet concrete enough to be relevant to and account for everyday situations.
4. Enable the user of the theory (practitioner) to have enough control over the everyday situations to make its application productive.

Wiedenbach sees the conceptual framework as dictating professional nursing practice as a service, provided to the individual with a need-for-help. The nursing action is purpose-directed, involving life, health, death, and the use of knowledge, judgment and skills.

Wiedenbach's model closely fits clinical nursing practice. Its focus clearly is the individual in need of help as a result of obstacles with which he/she is unable to cope independently. It applies to any situation that involves the professional practice of nursing since it defines the practice of nursing. It also allows flexibility for the practitioner to adapt methods as the circumstances change. This last point is important to a practice theory since, according to Wald and Leonard (1964) it "is not only limited to causal hypotheses but is further restricted to the use of causal variables that can be manipulated by the practitioner" (p 311). Wiedenbach's model provides for creativity by the practitioner in the manipulation of the environment or situation for the purpose of meeting the patient's need-for-help. An example of how Wiedenbach-based professional nursing practice would proceed is given below.

Practical Example:

Nurse interprets patient behavior.

Ms. Jones, R.N., enters Mrs. Smith's room. Mrs. Smith is one-day postcholesystectomy. Ms. Jones notes that Mrs. Smith grimaces as she changes her position. As she comes closer, she perceives beads of perspiration on Mrs. Smith's forehead. Ms. Jones decides to gather more information from Mrs. Smith about her perception of her condition.

Draws on knowledge.

Ms. Jones knows it would be consistent with usual recovery for a patient to be experiencing pain one day post-surgery. She checks her worksheet to note the time of Mrs. Smith's last analgesic which was 4½ hours ago.

Decision: Behavior inconsistent with comfort.

Ms. Jones: Mrs. Smith, you appear uncomfortable.

Mrs. Smith: I am. I was trying to change my positon to get more comfortable and in the process my stomach really started to hurt.

Obstacle: Condition; Seeks patient's perception, if need-for-help.

Ms. Jones: Do you mean your surgical site, or do you really mean your stomach?

Mrs. Smith: No, I mean from my surgery.

Ms. Jones: Is it severe enough that you would like some pain medication or has your change in position helped?

Patient unable to cope. Identification of need-for-help.

Mrs. Smith: Can I have something? It's really pretty bad, now.

Ms. Jones: Yes, I'll get it now.

Ministration

Ms. Jones leaves the room, returns with the medication and administers it. Twenty minutes later she returns to the room.

Validation

Ms. Jones: How are you feeling now Mrs. Smith?

Mrs. Smith: I'm feeling much better; that shot really helped.

Ms. Jones: Good. I'll check on you later.

Coordination of Resources

Ms. Jones goes to Mrs. Smith's chart and records the intervention and results.

SUMMARY

Wiedenbach's model appeared in a relatively early stage of theory development in nursing. It is one of the early attempts to systematically describe what it is that nurses do and what nursing is all about. Because of its strong inductive base it can be placed near the "abstracted empiricism" end of Merton's (1968) theoretical continuum.

As an earlier model, it is less clear in its definitions of the concepts of health and environment than the later models. It also does not clearly define one of the components, nursing art, in an operational way.

Its strengths lay in the focus of the model. It clearly focuses on the patient's perception of his/her conditions and, as such, is a significant nursing model because it is patient-centered (Ellis, 1968). Wiedenbach's model also takes a holistic view of man which is characteristic of professional nursing. It was written for the purpose of describing what takes place in the practice of professional nursing and here it succeeds very well. In summary, the Wiedenbach model is a significant contribution to the theoretical base of nursing.

REFERENCES

Abdellah FG: The nature of nursing science. Nursing Research, Vol 18, pp 300-392, 1969

Batey MV: Conceptualizing the research process. Nursing Research, Vol 20, pp 296-301, 1971

Berthold JS: Prologue. Nursing Research, Vol 17, pp 196-197, 1968

Blalock HM: Theory Construction. Prentice-Hall, Inc., Englewood Cliffs, New Jersey, 1969

Carper BA: Fundamental patterns of knowing in nursing. Advances in Nursing Science, Vol 1, No 1, pp 13-23, 1978

Dickoff J, James P: Researching research's role in theory development. Nursing Research, Vol 17, pp 204-206, 1968a

Dickoff J, James P: Theory of theories: A position paper. Nursing Research, Vol 17, pp 197-203, 1968b

Dubin R: Theory Building. The Free Press, New York, 1978

Duffey M, Muhlenkamp AF: A framework for theory analysis. Nursing Outlook, Vol 22, pp 570-574, 1974

Ellis R: Characteristics of significant theories. Nursing Research, Vol 17, No 3, pp 217-222, 1968

Fawcett J: The relationship between theory and research: A double helix. Advances in Nursing Science, Vol 1, No 1, pp 49-62, 1978

Glaser B, Strauss A: The Discovery of Grounded Theory. Aldine Publishing Co., Chicago, Illinois, 1967

Hardy ME (ed): Theoretical Foundations for Nursing. MSS Information Corporation, New York, 1973

Hardy ME: Theories: Components, development, evaluation. Nursing Research, Vol 23, pp 100-107, 1974

Hardy ME: Perspectives on nursing theory. Advances in Nursing Science, Vol 1, No 1, pp 37-48, 1978

Jacox A: Theory construction in nursing: An overview. Nursing Research, Vol 23, pp 4-13, 1974

Johnson DE: Theory in nursing: Borrowed and unique. Nursing Research, Vol 17, pp 206-209, 1968

Merton RK: Social Theory and Social Structure. The Free Press, New York, 1968

Rudner RS: Philosophy of social sciences. Prentice-Hall, Inc. Englewood Cliffs, New Jersey, 1966-1967

Wald FS, Leonard RC: Toward development of practice theory. Nursing Research, Vol 13, pp 309-313, 1964

Walker LO: Toward a clearer understanding of the concept of nursing theory. Nursing Research, Vol 20, pp 428-435, 1971

Wiedenbach E: Clinical Nursing: A Helping Art. Springer, New York, 1964

6

HENDERSON'S DEFINITION
OF NURSING

Judith Aumente Runk & Stephanie I. Muth Quillin

INTRODUCTION

Virginia Henderson received her first preparation in nursing at the Army School of Nursing in Washington which she entered in 1921. After a brief career as a staff nurse, she began teaching at Norfolk Protestant Hospital. Five years later, she entered Teacher's College, Columbia University, where she earned a B.S. and M.A. in nursing education. She rejoined the Teacher's College faculty in 1930 and remained there until 1948 where she taught courses in clinical practice and the analytical process. In 1953, she worked with Leo Simmons on a national survey of nursing research. In 1959, she directed the *Nursing Studies Index* project through Yale University. The *Nursing Studies Index* was composed of four volumes of the analytical, historical, and biographical literature on nursing from 1900 to 1959. This index demonstated that a body of literature in nursing was inaccessible through existing indexes and was influential in the publication of the *International Nursing Index* (Safier, 1977).

In 1981, Henderson advised new graduate nurses to develop and enrich themselves through the arts, sciences, and humanities; to be involved in local, national, and worldwide affairs; and, to study the art as well as the science of nursing (McCarty, 1981). In her writings, Henderson (1966) presents a definition of nursing based on her personal understandings. While her work does not fall into what may be strictly interpreted as a theory of nursing, analysis shows it to be in an important pre-paradigm stage.

In her writings, Henderson cites those who influenced her work. Annie Goodrich, as director of the Army School of Nursing, influenced Henderson's understandings of the concept of patient-centered care. At Teacher's College, Columbia University, Henderson was exposed to the work of Stackpole in cell physiology and Thorndike in psychology. The philosophy of Tielhard de Chardin introduced Henderson to ideas of the increasing complexity of life. Henderson refers to her debt to Orlando (1961) and Weidenbach (1964). Orlando's influence is seen in Henderson's statement that the nurse must be aware of the nonverbal communications of patients. Henderson also refers to the ability of the nurse to act on patient needs after she/he has confirmed the accurate meaning of behavior with the patients (1966). Weidenbach (1964) clarified the deliberative nursing approach for Henderson (1966). The deliberative approach supported Henderson's belief that the worker is influenced by his/her goals. It might appear that Orem's (1980) concept of self-care is related to Henderson's definition of nursing. Orem's work, however, makes no specific mention of Henderson's influence.

BASIC CONSIDERATIONS
INCLUDED IN THE MODEL

Henderson views nursing as an independent, unique health profession. It is a profession which requires university education, conducts research, and enjoys a collegial relationship with the other health-related professions (1955, 1961). The four concepts of person, nursing, health, and environment are found within Henderson's definition, either implicitly or explicitly.

Definitions of Nursing, Person, Health, and Environment

Nursing is defined in terms of its function. "The unique function of the nurse is to assist the individual, sick or well, in performance of those activities contributing to health or its recovery (or peaceful death) that he/she would perform unaided if he/she had the necessary strength, will or knowledge. And to do this in such a way as to help him/her gain independence as rapidly as possible" (Henderson, p 15, 1966).

According to Henderson, persons are biological beings whose mind and body are inseparable. She views physical and emotional balance as based on fluctuations and responses in cellular physiology. Each person has fundamental needs for shelter, food, and communication. Further, persons must have the company of loved ones, the opportunity to win approval, to learn, to work, to play and to worship. Despite these commonalities, each individual is unique in the way that these needs are operationalized (Henderson, 1966).

Henderson believes health is basic to human functioning. The definition of health is viewed as the individual's ability to function independently in relation to the 14 components of basic nursing care (Henderson, 1966). These 14 components are:

1. Breathe normally.
2. Eat and drink adequately.
3. Eliminate body waste.
4. Move and maintain desirable postures.
5. Sleep and rest.
6. Select suitable clothes—dress and undress.
7. Maintain body temperature within normal range by adjusting clothing and modifying the environment.
8. Keep the body clean and well groomed and protect the integument.
9. Avoid changes in the environment and avoid injuring others.
10. Communicate with others expressing emotions, needs, fears or opinions.
11. Worship according to one's faith.
12. Work in such a way that there is a sense of accomplishment.
13. Play or participate in various forms of recreation.
14. Learn, discover, or satisfy the curiosity that leads to normal development and health and use the available health facilities (Henderson, pp 16-17, 1966).

Completeness and wholeness of mind and body are viewed by Henderson as a rarely achieved state of health (1966). Health is equated with independence on a continuum that has illness equated with dependence. The definition of health as conceived by the World Health Organization (WHO) is seen by Henderson as a valid goal (1966). That definition states that "... health is a state of complete physical, mental and social well-being, not merely the absence of disease or infirmity" (World Health Organization, p 29, 1947). This definition was revolutionary in its time although it has now been criticized because of its myriad social and political implications as well as the impossibility of objectively attaining or even defining such a state.

Environment is not clearly defined. Henderson agrees with Nightingale, who sees nature as the real nurturer and curer. The nurse acts as the intermediary between person and the environment (Henderson, 1966). Henderson lists seven health essentials in the environment: light, temperature, air movement, atmospheric pressure, appropriate disposal of waste, minimal quantities of injurious chemicals, and cleanliness of surfaces and furnishings coming in contact with the individual. She devotes a chapter in the text, *Principles and Practices of Nursing,* to "Organization and Care of the Environment." Henderson recognizes that the environment can act upon the patient in either a positive or negative way. It is, therefore, the function of the nurse to alter the environment in such a way as to support the patient. The definitions of person, health, and nursing emphasize individualized care, family-centered care, and rehabilitation (Harmer & Henderson, 1955).

Description of Nursing Activity or the Nursing Process

Henderson's conceptualization of nursing is based on a dimension of practice. Much of this practice is seen as linked to a hospital. Henderson documents the need for an individualized plan of care. In many ways this is seen as the precursor of nursing process and nursing diagnosis. Nursing activities which recognize the patient's needs and wants, and which are "individualized," are to be documented in a written format.

Nursing action, according to Henderson, is deliberative, i.e., planned, executed, and evaluated. Each of the 14 components of nursing care is to be assessed and prioritized. Individualized care, i.e., care which recognizes the uniqueness of the patient and the nurse, is designed, administered, and documented for further evaluation and assessment.

Henderson states that the patient's needs must be validated with her/him and the effectiveness of nursing measures confirmed. The patient actively participates in his/her care. Patient teaching is a critical activity for the patient who lacks "sufficient knowledge." The nurse assumes activities for the patient which she/he cannot do for her/himself. The nurse allows and encourages the patient to be independent through performance of the 14 basic components. The deliberateness of nursing activity coupled with the importance of evaluating and documenting the care given predate the formal development of nursing process.

Understanding of Person

Henderson sees persons as biological beings whose mind and body are inseparable. It is here that we see the influence of Stackpole and Thorndike. The emphasis on cellular physiology represents the clearest thinking at the time of Henderson's nursing definition. The definition of fundamental needs reflects the explorations in psychology in the 1950s. Persons are seen as integrated wholes by Thorndike and Maslow. The 14 components of basic nursing care and the definition of nursing extended Thorndike's research in psychology to the patient in the hospital. Henderson explored how the person's need for shelter and food was met when she/he assumed the role of patient. Henderson's person is heavily biologically-oriented. The 14 basic needs are weighted towards biological needs. Through Stackpole at Columbia University, Henderson integrated the concept of balance, both physiological and behavioral.

Understanding of Health

Health is equated with independence in Henderson's definition. The 14 nursing care components are aimed toward moving the patient from a state of varying degrees of dependence imposed by illness to a state of independence. Implicit in this understanding of health is the realization that persons make choices about their state of health and while the nurse can facilitate these choices, the ultimate responsibility for health is borne by the person.

Interrelationships Between the Concepts

Nursing is defined by its function, according to Henderson. The nurse plans care appropriate to "assisting the individual" in activities contributing to his/her health. When coupled with the 14 care concepts, one can see that the nurse cares for the patient in a patient-centered way. Figure 6.1 shows the interrelationships of person, nursing, and the environment in Henderson's conceptualization of nursing.

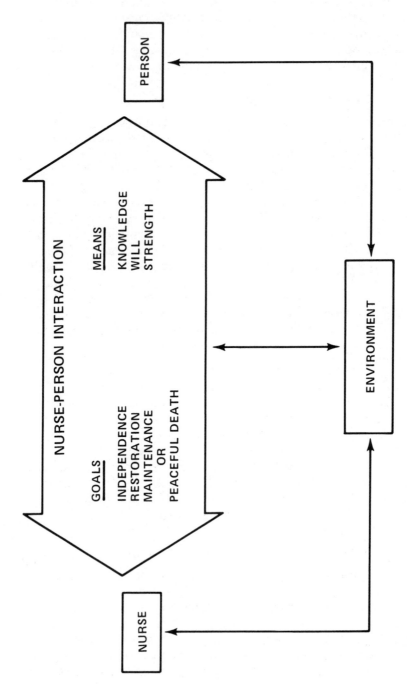

Figure 6.1. Interrelationship of Person, Nursing, and Environment.

The definition of nursing by Henderson states functions of nursing and develops the activities apropriate to nursing. Person, nursing, and health are related in that the nurse attempts to operationalize these concepts into patient-centered care.

INTERNAL ANALYSIS

Underlying Assumptions

Henderson bases her definition of nursing on several implicit assumptions. They are:

1. Independence is valued by the nurse and the patient more than dependence.
2. Health has a meaning shared by the society at large.
3. Individuals desire health or a peaceful death and will act in such a way as to achieve this.
4. Individuals will perform activities leading to health if they have the knowledge, capacity, or will.
5. The individual's goals and the nurse's goals are congruent.
6. The 14 basic needs represent nursing's basic functions.
7. Nursing's goals may be subsumed into the medical treatment plan.

The major explicit assumption is Henderson's contention that the nurse is an independent practitioner and as such is the authority on basic nursing care. She also states that the nurse acts as the physician's prime helper in carrying out physician's prescriptions (Henderson, 1966). In this respect she indirectly supports the stereotyped role of the nurse.

The relationship between the explicit and implicit assumption is an interesting one. The values and assumptions implied in the model are those of nursing and its relationship to the health and well-being of the client. It is assumed that it is the interaction between nurse and patient that results in health. However, the explicit assumptions are inconsistent with the characteristics of a profession in that Henderson contends that the nurse as an independent professional acts with and for the physician, another professional.

Central Components of the Model

Henderson's definition of nursing sees person as having biological, sociological and spirtual components. These components are operationalized in the 14 basic needs. A second major component of the definition is that of nursing function, and the third component is the interaction of the two of these in the process called nursing care. The components of nursing and person have been previously defined. Figure 6.1 represents the interaction of these elements. This interaction results in the uniqueness of nursing practice. Henderson believes that although there are a limited number of basic human needs, there are infinite ways of meeting those needs (Henderson, 1961).

Henderson places the individual in a primary position in her definition. Nursing acts in relation to that individual. In some instances it seems that the nurse in Henderson's definition keeps blinders on in relation to society and to the impact that society has on the health of the individual. Henderson's definition of nursing and the 14 basic needs are stated in such a way as to imply that persons respond without any influence from society or their families. However, her later writings recognize the importance and variability of these resources.

Health and the restoration of health as it relates to the individual is ranked next in importance. The nurse's importance is based on her ability to define the needs of the client and assist him/her rationally in meeting these needs.

The units of Henderson's definition are summative units (Dubin, 1978). Summative units represent the entire complex of a thing, in this case, nursing. Numerous properties of the thing are drawn together and the label given them emphasizes the common elements. The summative nature of the unit limits the theory-building potential of Henderson's model.

Henderson's definition of nursing consists of a description of nursing functions and application of those functions to practice, research, and education. This description fits the pre-paradigm stage of theory development. At the pre-paradigm stage, a theory is very readable and provides a perspective rather than a set of interrelated theoretical statements. The terms are ill-defined but have meanings close to everyday language (Hardy, 1978). All of this is apparent within Henderson's definition. Henderson uses theoretical positions from psychology and physiology in her needs statements. She builds her definition from elements in other areas. What she develops is not exclusively nursing but when put together in a certain configuration, becomes nursing.

Henderson's definitions can be assessed by some of the criteria used for analyzing theory. It can be assessed for its meaning and logical adequacy and its operational and empirical adequacy (Hardy, 1974). It can also be assessed in terms of its scope, complexity and usefulness as well as its ability to generate information (Ellis, 1968).

Logical adequacy is assessed by looking at Henderson's implicit assumptions. The implicit assumptions, particularly those which emphasize independence and the universality of the meaning of health, are inconsistent with the literature on illness behavior. Practitioners have seen that health may be perceived differently by individual clients. These perceptions may be vastly different from those of the nurse. The explicit assumption which places the nurse in a supportive position of the physician is inconsistent with generally held definitions that point to the unique function and independence of professionals. This explicit requirement to support the physician limits the applicability of the model.

Because Henderson's constructs are summative units, it is not possible to directly delineate hypotheses from them. Henderson says what "is" from her personal viewpoint of nursing. Henderson's definition of nursing and the basic needs have the scope to affect both nursing theory and nursing practice. The definition of nursing relates to persons sick or well who need the services of the nurse to assist in activities she/he would do had she/he the knowledge and will. The basic needs include more physiological parameters than social, cultural, or spiritual. Although Henderson's definition has the potential to encompass the whole person, in fact the definition of nursing is limited primarily to physiological parameters.

Complexity is present in this definition of nursing. However, the nursing definition needs further theoretical development. The basic needs appear simple; however, any attempt to alter, for example, nutrition patterns is complex when all the parameters of this need are considered.

Henderson's perspective of nursing has guided clinical practice through the widespread use of the textbook, *Principles and Practices of Nursing* (Harmer & Henderson, 1955). The frequency with which the needs are referenced when practitioners document nursing care is further evidence of Henderson's influence. In this respect Henderson's model has turned out to be a useful although somewhat limited nursing model.

Henderson generated the elements of other conceptual models. For example, the Nursing Development Conference Group (Orem, 1979) uses components of Henderson's definition to evolve the concept of nursing agency. While this reference is never specifically made, it is possible that Henderson's definition of nursing and of the 14 basic needs are implicit as a part of nursing understandings.

Henderson's definition of nursing served the practice of nursing well. It broadened the function of nursing and was specific enough to differentiate nursing from other professions. It described a profession which needed to be university-based and engaged in research. This definition has been built upon extensively by nursing in the development of the scientific discipline through theory development, research, and professional practice.

EXTERNAL THEORY ANALYSIS

Relationships to Nursing Research

Henderson philosophically and practically supports the concept of nursing research. She states:

"Unless one believes in the born nurse or in the assumption that a nurse acts under the orders of the physician who will design the methods she uses, there seems to be no reason why she should not subject her practice to the same type of analysis that characterizes all comparable occupations." (Henderson, p 33, 1966)

Henderson is opposed to studies about the characteristics of nurses or time-motion studies that characterized nursing's early research base. Henderson sees research as being the most fruitful method for decision-making in nursing. She defines research as "a structured systematic investigation designed to answer a question, throw light on a theory, or solve a problem " (Henderson, p 33, 1966). Henderson's examples of research questions call for applied or prescriptive level research. However, her definition of research implies that all levels of nursing research are appropriate.

If the 14 basic needs define the scope of nursing practice, then research questions arise from them. For example, what postoperative positions decrease pain; what kinds of teaching plans are effective in improving nutrition of the obese patient; how may commonly used equipment be altered in design for patient comfort? Henderson was one of the earliest thinkers in nursing to recognize the need for a written, individualized plan of care (Henderson, 1966). This precursor of nursing process provided documentation for the activities of the nurse. These care plans give practitioners a sense of what the recurring needs of the patient are and suggest nursing interventions to meet these needs.

Relationships To Nursing Education

Henderson organized a curriculum around basic needs and symptoms found within the patient. The final course of study focuses on disease-oriented nursing (Henderson, 1966). This organization represents an attempt to move away from the medical model. The textbook, *Principles and Practices of Nursing*, in which the definition of nursing is found, was revised in 1978 and has been used as a basic text in many schools of nursing. It provides a view of nursing that introduces the beginning student to the values of the profession. This is an appropriate use of a model composed of summative units (Dubin, 1978).

Henderson states that the only place a nurse can be educated in this country and meet the criteria of independence and creative thinking is in a college or university. This statement post-dates the 1965 American Nurses Association Position on Nursing and supports the earlier work of Brown (1948) and Russell (1958). The official ANA position as well as the earlier commissioned studies by Brown and Russell supported the view that education for the professional practice of nursing should take place in institutions of higher education.

Henderson's Teacher's College background is evident in her work. Her curriculum models speak of structured learning experiences that are goal-directed. The nurse, after the initial program of learning, is a generalist. Further education allows for specialization. This concept is in keeping with professional education in other professional fields.

If graduate nurses are to function independently, then student nurses must be taught in non-regimented creative ways. Henderson believes that the student should have input into his/her curriculum in much the same way as the patient has input into his/her care. Her beliefs reflect the influence of John Dewey and Teacher's College. It is important to remember that Henderson was operationalizing this philosophy at a time when nursing education was very regimented.

Henderson's curriculum designs provide a source for educational research. The ideas inherent in them, e.g., that the nursing student is not a worker and that nursing school faculty should provide models for professional practitioners, were considered revolutionary. These ideas reflect Henderson's values. While they are not necessarily shared by other nursing leaders, they no longer seem revolutionary. It is possible that Henderson's definition might guide an educational program in today's social and political times, but it is unlikely that this will occur. The statements she makes seem far too general to provide a guide to curriculum development.

Relationship to Nursing Practice

Henderson's definition of nursing relates to nursing as a practice discipline. She succinctly states that:

"We want to provide for a man's universal needs but with infinite modifications in nursing care according to the ever unique requirements of the individual." (Henderson, p 42, 1966)

Direct service in the form of direct care to the patient is rewarding insofar as the nurse can help the patient toward independence. However, Henderson is vague about the "social rewards." This definition was written in the 1960s, an era on the American political scene that brought a new awareness of social and political inequities. Her definition would be strengthened by greater recognition of the social upheaval taking place. The first stirrings of the consumer health movement were being heard but there is no mention of this activism. The 14 basic needs are reflective of physiological changes. They show little recognition of complex psychosocial or cultural needs. For example, sexuality is not discussed. Appreciation and support of culturally proscribed health beliefs is not mentioned. The role that nursing has played in supporting the physician has limited nursing's credibility with the women's movement.

Henderson contributes a deliberative, decision-making approach to patient-care. This approach has relevance today as nurses routinely use the steps of nursing process in their practice. Documented plans of care now exist as a permanent part of the patient's record. It is now possible to collect data about nursing practice and to develop quantitative research questions from this qualitative data.

Henderson recognizes the person as a complex being who interacts with the environment. This is a strength of her conceptual effort. The nurse makes individualized plans with the health team for both short-term and long-term needs. Dependency is seen as an important period in patient care, but one which the nurse seeks to shorten. The weakness of the definition lies in its lack of generalizability to different social or cultural aspects of the patient or nurse. For example, in some cultures, the appropriate role for the sick person is one of dependence, with the family providing nursing care.

SUMMARY

Henderson's definition of nursing, which includes the 14 basic needs, was a valuable contribution to the discipline of nursing. She did not claim that it was a model of nursing; however, it contains some of the elements of a model. More importantly, it articulates a value system that has had an impact on practice, research, and education. Its strengths lie in the use of a deliberate approach in the delivery of care and a view of the person as a complex bio-psychosocial being. The curriculum for nursing education that it generates is based on the liberal arts.

The summative nature of its concepts limits its use in theory building. This definition acted as a stimulus to other, more formally developed theories. Henderson may best be described as a quiet revolutionary in the field of nursing. She practiced her beliefs about nursing in education, research, and professional practice, and influenced the practice of nursing around the world.

REFERENCES

Brown EL: Nursing for the Future. Russell Sage Foundation, New York, 1948

Dubin R: Theory Building. The Free Press, New York, 1978

Ellis R: Characteristics of significant theories. Nursing Research, Vol 17, No 3, pp 217-222, 1968

Hardy M: Theories: Components, development, evaluation. Nursing Research, Vol 23, pp 100-107, 1974

Hardy M: Perspectives on nursing theory. Advances in Nursing Science, Vol 1, pp 37-48, 1978

Harmer B, Henderson V: Textbook of the Principles and Practice of Nursing, 5th ed. Macmillan Company, New York, 1955

Henderson V: The Nature of Nursing: A Definition and Its Implications, Practice, Research, and Education. Macmillan Company, New York, 1966

Henderson V: Basic Principles of Nursing Care. International Council of Nurses, Geneva, Switzerland, 1972

McCarty P: Notable nurses, friends offer advice to graduates. The American Nurse, Vol 13, No 5, 1981

Orem DE (ed): Concept Formalization in Nursing: Process and Product. Little, Brown & Co., Boston, Massachusetts, 1979

Orem DE: Nursing: Concepts of practice, 2nd ed. McGraw-Hill Book Co., New York, 1980

Orlando IJ: The Dynamic Nurse-Patient Relationship, Function, Process and Principles. G.P. Putnam's Sons, New York, 1961

Russell CH: Liberal education and nursing. Nursing Research, Vol 7, pp 116-126, 1958

Safier G: Contemporary American Leaders in Nursing: An Oral History. McGraw-Hill Book Co., New York, 1977

Weidenbach E: Clinical Nursing: A Helping Art. Springer Publishing Co., New York, 1964

World Health Organization: Geneva, Switzerland, 1947

7

LEVINE'S NURSING MODEL

Barbara A. Pieper

INTRODUCTION

During the 1960s and 1970s, three types of theory-building efforts were evident in nursing, i.e., the use of borrowed theory, an effort to develop practice theory, and development of nursing conceptual models. In 1962 the federal government began to fund the nurse-scientist program, in large part for the purpose of developing nurse-scientists who might develop nursing's theoretical base. Knowledge from varied disciplines was thus used to build the scientific base of nursing. Practice or practical theory was identified during this time as the systematic study of the nursing experience. A major difficulty with development of practice theory was a lack of agreement regarding a definition of nursing (Newman, 1972). When the nursing conceptual models such as Rogers' were developed and presented, a conceptual system of nursing with the person identified as the center of nursing's purpose (Newman, 1972) was begun. Much of the emphasis upon practice theory began to wane. The person was often seen in the models as a bio-psychosocial being and nursing, it was decided, emphasized this holism.

Although she had prior journal publications, Levine's model of nursing was published in 1969 in *An Introduction to Nursing.* Levine's work is reflective of all three types of theory-building efforts noted above. Levine borrowed knowledge from the basic sciences, e.g., psychology, sociology, and physiology, used this knowledge to analyze varied nursing practice situations and described in some detail nursing skills and activities. Levine's nursing activity analyses resulted in the formulation of her model, which is divided into nine models. She considered these models to be a structural framework for understanding a wide variety of related nursing processes. Finally, Levine presented the "person" in a holistic manner and as the center of nursing activity. The "person" in Levine's model is the ill individual in a health care setting. Emphasis on the ill person in the health care setting is also reflective of the history of health care of the 1960s when the person, more often than not, is seen as ill and hospitalized. Thus Levine developed a model of nursing which reflects the historical evolutionary nursing theory. It should also be noted that Levine's model was developed for beginning students of nursing. Consideration of historical placement of Levine's model should be made when present day model analysis systems are used. That is, Levine's model is not as fully developed nor should it be expected to be as well developed as later models. Her work made possible many of the later speculations regarding the nature of person, environment, health and nursing.

ANALYSIS OF BASIC CONSIDERATIONS

A nursing model can be considered a perspective for examining nursing; it is descriptive. Concepts common to all nursing models are the definitions and consideration of person, environment, health, and nursing.

Definition of Person

Person is not defined as such in Levine's model, but indeed the person as the object of nursing care is discussed in all of her writings. The person is presented as a complex individual who interacts with environment. The individual is continuous with the environment and is characterized by an incessant exchange of information which is absolutely necessary for survival (Levine, 1971). Emphasizing adaptation, Levine (1971) further states that the person is a living being in interaction with environment, responding to change in an orderly, sequential pattern, and thus adapting and adapted to the forces which shape and reshape the essence of the person. Successful interaction of the person with environment so as to conserve or defend self or wholeness depends upon a regulatory system, specifically the nervous system

(Levine, 1973). Unordered and unregulated change in the person is considered disruptive of life and results in disease and subsequently death.

Definition of Environment

In Levine's approach, each individual has both an internal and an external environment. The internal environment is represented in nursing by the study of physiology and pathophysiology (Levine, p 12, 1973). Levine's definition of external environment was borrowed from Bates (1967). External environment relates to factors which impinge upon and change the individual. External environment has the following components:

1. Perceptual—aspects of the environment responded to with the sense organs
2. Operational—factors in the environment which cannot be perceived by the sense organs, e.g., radioactivity and micro-organisms
3. Conceptual—factors which affect human behavior, e.g., language, value systems, religion, traditions

The environmental setting which Levine presents for the nurse-patient interaction is the hospital. However, she does recognize the importance of larger social systems, i.e., education, employment, as well as the community-at-large with its resources, attitudes, and a certain commitment to health care (Levine, p 18, 1973). Since the nurse is employed by the hospital, is with the patient the greatest amount of time, and explains various rules and procedures to the patient, the nurse represents the image of the hospital to the patient (Levine, p 31, 1973). In the hospital environment, the nurse must learn to work with illness, anxiety, fear, and pain in a therapeutic manner. Although the hospital is an artificial environment, Levine stressed that nursing with its scientific principles and holistic concept of the person is learned at the bedside.

Definition of Health

Levine (1973) defined health in terms of the Anglo-Saxon word meaning "whole" (p 11). With growth and development, the changing patterns of response to the environment create changing dimensions of wholeness for the individual (Levine, p 157,

1971). Health and disease are patterns of adaptive change. Disease represents an effort of the individual to protect self integrity, i.e., the inflammatory response (Levine, p 257, 1971). All forces influencing a person's response to illness do not exist as discrete activities but as dynamic relationships seeking an equilibrium for uniformity of function (Levine, p 2452, 1970).

Levine defines and presents the concepts of health and disease in an historic and anthropologic manner. Levine (1973) states that every society has means to care for the ill and, as emphasized by Nightingale, nature was the first healer. The germ theory resulted in care being focused on the disease, often with the patient as a person totally ignored. Finally, the behavioral sciences drew attention to the multiple factors of disease; recognition of psychosocial needs of the individual resulted in nursing exploring "total patient care" (Levine, 1973).

Definition of Nursing

Levine defines nursing as a human interaction—an exchange between individuals. Nursing is a subculture, possessing ideas and values which are unique to nurses and which reflect society. Nursing knowledge allows for a sensitive and productive relationship between the nurse and the individual needing care (Levine, p 1, 1973). Reflecting borrowed knowledge, nursing practice thus follows the prevaling theories of health and disease.

Through the nursing process, Levine presents a description of nursing activity. Concepts of the nursing process are many and include the following:

1. "The nurse participates actively in every patient's environment, and much of what she does supports his adjustments as he struggles in the predicament of illness" (Levine, p 2452, 1970).
2. "Decisions for nursing intervention must be based on the unique behavior of the individual patient" (Levine, p 2452, 1970).
3. "(Individualized) nursing intervention can take place only when the nurse has made an accurate assessment of the (individual's) unique needs, and this in turn is possible only through the formulation of all relevant factors that contribute to the patient's predicament at a given time and place" (Levine, p 23, 1973).

4. "With nursing intervention, the nurse interposes her skills and knowledge into the course of events that affect the patient" (Levine, p 13, 1973).

Levine, as did Nightingale, placed great emphasis on observation. Observation allows the nurse to evaluate the patient's condition as well as anticipate the patient's future course of events. An important dimension in observation is the passage of time. Observations are continuous, repetitive, and changing (Levine, p 24, 1973). Since observations are a tool for directing patient care, observations must be shared, e.g., nurse-to-physician or nurse-to-nurse.

Evolving her concept for nursing process, Levine added a discussion of nursing diagnosis in her 1973 model. A diagnosis provides direction and influences the kinds of examinations and therapies which may be selected to treat a patient (Levine, p 26, 1973). An advantage of a diagnosis is the language which is universally understood and which transmits information in a few words. Levine does differentiate a medical diagnosis from a nursing diagnosis. Since nursing diagnosis was historically a new term and poorly understood, Levine (1973) recommended that the nurse use steps of the scientific method for establishing of guidelines for patient care (p 29). The assessment process of nursing and rationale for nursing intervention are highly emphasized in Levine's model, although her model accentuates nursing intervention. Nursing intervention occurs only when the nurse has made an accurate assessment of needs through formulation of all relevant factors that contribute to the patient's situation (Levine, p 23, 1973).

Since an illness threatens life space, the person with an illness comes to the nurse (Levine, p 211, 1970). The person as a patient does have a role in the health care environment, but Levine depicts the patient mainly as ill and dependent. However, the nurse-patient relationship is seen as an important and dynamic one in which each participant must recognize the strengths of the other (Levine, p 2106, 1970).

Summary of Basic Considerations

Levine does discuss the concepts of person, environment, health, and nursing. Nursing is a human interaction between individuals and for which nursing has an extant body of knowledge. The person is complex in nature and interacts with the environment. The nurse-patient interaction mainly occurs in the hospital where the patient is ill, dependent, and in an unfamiliar environment. The nurse uses the nursing process, i.e., assessment, intervention, and evaluation when interacting with the patient. The nurse is the primary person in the hospital environment. The interaction of the basic concepts of Levine's model are presented in Figure 7.1. All persons possess an internal and external environment. Components of the external environment are perceptual, operational, and conceptual. The person is seen primarily as dependent. The nurse and patient interact usually in the hospital setting and although the patient participates in care, the nurse is the primary force. Conservation is the maintenance of the proper balance between nursing interventions and patient participation. Holistic care thus can result from consideration of all of these components.

INTERNAL ANALYSIS OF A MODEL

When examining internal model components, one should consider definitions, concepts, assumptions, propositions, and model building efforts. Major definitions of person, nursing, health, and environment have previously been presented. The following section will explore Levine's model as to concepts, assumptions, propositions, and model-building efforts and will present an example of each. No internal theory components are explicitly stated by Levine.

Concepts

Dubin (1978) defines a concept as a unit and identifies units as the things out of which theories are built (p 28). Concepts are also mental images; they are defined within a theory (Popper, 1963; Hardy, 1974). Concepts may be operationally or abstractly defined. Two major concepts in Levine's model are holism and adaptation. With holism, Levine integrates the major definitions of man, nursing, health, and environment. Levine (1973) states that the life process of the organism is dependent upon the interrelatedness of component systems (p 8). Levine (1973) notes that the word holistic is derived from *hol* which means entire (p 12). Holism recognizes an open, constantly changing interaction of the individual with the internal and external environment. Holism emphasizes the need for nursing to individualize care to each patient's assessment. Holism also encompasses Levine's

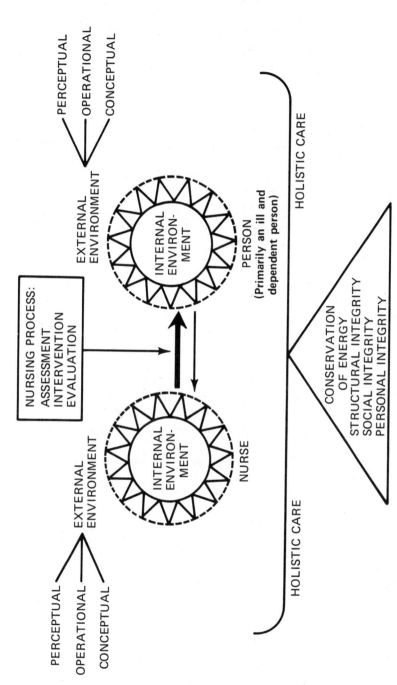

Figure 7.1. Representation of Person, Health, Environment, and Nursing in Levine's Model.

(1973) definition of health derived from *hal* meaning whole (p 11).
In the last chapter of her model, Levine (1973) presents the
dimension of the holistic response which integrates the environment, psychophysiology, and consideration of biorhythms.

Levine (1973) states that adaptation is the process of change;
survival depends upon the quality of adaptation possible for the
individual. Integrating basic model components, Levine (1973)
states that health and disease are patterns of adaptive change. By
participating in the individual's environment, the nurse supports
the person's adaptation. All adaptation represents accommo-
dation between the internal and external envirnoment. The
individual's ability to adapt influences nursing intervention. If
adaptation is directed toward social well-being, then nursing
interventions are therapeutic; if adaptation is directed toward
maintenance of status quo or a downward course, then nursing
interventions are supportive (Levine, p 13, 1973).

Assumptions

Assumptions can be viewed as relational statements which
are accepted as truths and, as such, are not tested (Abdellah,
1969). Examples of Levine's assumptions are:
1. Person—Since person is not explicitly defined by Levine,
   assumptions about the person are integrated with other
   concepts. "Erikson has described wholeness as an open
   system. He writes, '...The unceasing interaction of the
   individual organism with its environments does represent an *open and fluid* system"*..." (Levine, p 11, 1973).
2. Nursing—"The nurse provides care for that patient"
   (Levine, p 27, 1973).
3. Health—"Health and disease are patterns of adaptive
   change" (Levine, p 11, 1973).
4. Environment—"The nurse participates actively in every
   patient's environment... (Levine, p 13, 1973).

Assumptions may be explicitly or implicitly stated in a
theory but since Levine did not label statements as assumptions,
Levine's assumptions are thought to be implicit.

Propositions

Propositions are concerned with predictions about the value
of units in the system; they are truth statements that may be
made about a theoretical model (Dubin, p 165, 1969). Dubin

*Erikson E: Identity: Youth and Crisis. W.W. Norton and Co., Inc., New York,
1968

(1969) continues that "there is no logic by which the truth statements about one model may be brought into congruence with those of a different model" (p 167). Levine's major propositions are the four principles of conservation. Conservation is a maintenance of a proper balance between active nursing intervention coupled with patient participation. The four principles of conservation are:

1. Principle of the conservation of energy.
   The individual's ability to function is dependent upon energy balance, i.e., the supply of nutrients measured against the rate of energy expenditure.
2. Principle of the conservation of structural integrity.
   The process of healing is the process of restoration of structural integrity. "Structural change results in a change in function, and pathophysiological processes all present a threat to structural integrity" (Levine, p 50, 1967).
3. Principle of the conservation of personal integrity.
   Individuals respond to illness in a personal manner. Since self identity and self respect are the foundations of personal integrity, important to the ill person are privacy, participation in decision-making, consent of treatment, teaching, and confidentiality of knowledge (Levine, p 54, 1967).
4. Principle of the conservation of social integrity.
   Even though hospitalized and ill, an individual needs social contact such as from family, religion, and the community. An individual knows self in the reflection of others (Levine, p 56, 1967). If family and friends are included in the patient's care, the nurse gains an understanding of the person in a social network.

Consistent with her definitions, Levine's propositions emphasize the ill, hospitalized individual, the importance of nursing assessment, and provision of nursing skills. The propositions are stated early in her model and are consistent throughout the model.

Model Building

Models are symbolic representations of perceptual phenomena and vary in abstraction (McKay, p 394, 1969). Pictorial models attempt to reproduce the important features of an event for the purpose of making possible closer scrutiny and manipulation (McKay, p 394, 1969). Levine (1973) uses pictorial models such as a negative feedback system and positive feedback system diagrams.

Descriptive models represent the structure of the relationship within the reality setting (McKay, p 394, 1969). Levine outlines nine descriptive models. Each model emphasizes beginning level pathophysiology and psychosocial content specific to that model. Levine also allows for understanding and application of her model in a broad spectrum of disease conditions. The nine models and the biopsychosocial content presented in each are the following:

1. Vital signs—biopsychosocial concepts of temperature, pulse, and respiration (Levine, 1973).
2. Body movement and positioning—biopsychosocial concepts of body mechanics, patient positioning, and bedrest (Levine, 1973).
3. Ministration of personal hygiene needs—biopsychosocial concepts of personal hygiene, medical asepsis, and integumentary assessment (Levine, 1973).
4. Pressure gradient systems in nursing intervention (fluids)—biopsychosocial concepts of fluids and pressure gradients (Levine, 1973).
5. Nursing determinants in provision for nutritional needs—biopsychosocial concepts of foods and diet therapy (Levine, 1973).
6. Pressure gradient systems in nursing (gases)—biopsychosocial concepts of respiratory function (Levine, 1973).
7. Local application of heat and cold—biopsychosocial concepts of heat and cold (Levine, 1973).
8. Administration of medications—biopsychosocial concepts of drug administration (Levine, 1973).
9. Establishing an aseptic environment—biopsychosocial concepts of microorganisms, infection, and aseptic technique (Levine, 1973).

Each model emulates from the previously presented biophysical content and conservation of energy principles for a patient problem. For example, model 6, pressure gradient systems in nursing (gas exchange), follows content on nursing the patient with a disturbance of homeostasis in systemic oxygen needs. It is interesting that Levine did not develop a descriptive model for the content section emphasizing holistic care, a major concept in her writings. These models are also an example of deductive scientific argument.

Models vary in terms of the metaphor—machine or organism—that is used (McKay, p 394, 1969). An open, self-maintaining and self-regulating biological system is an organismic model. Whereas a machine model would view man as an inert instrument performing assigned tasks, Levine's models are organismic as demonstrated by the concepts of holism and nurse-patient interaction.

Summary and Evaluation of Internal Analysis

Ellis (1968) states that the purpose of theory is to order facts, structure facts from other fields, give direction to practice, and assist in retrieval of information. Levine borrowed concepts from other fields and attempted to order them in regard to nursing. The person she presents, though, is the ill, hospitalized patient as evidenced by the word "patient" throughout her writing. Although emphasis is placed on physiology, psychosocial factors are integrated throughout her model, thus demonstrating complexity of multiple variables. Scope of the model is limited due to the emphasis on the ill person. Since Levine's descriptive model was written as a fundamental nursing textbook, it had usefulness in assisting the beginning student to organize principles of assessment and skills in a nursing framework. Implicit values were recognized and made explicit as evidenced by her early statement of holistic man and subsequent integration of bio-psychosocial content into her nine models.

Johnson (1974) presents three evaluative guides for nursing theory—social congruence, social significance, and social unity. Levine's model is socially congruent since it is based on expectations of society that a person is a holistic being and that nursing care assists the individual to adapt. Social significance, or the effect of outcomes in making a difference on the level of well-being, is questionable in Levine's model since nursing is emphasized in a hospital environment. The social significance of the individual in the community and family or the role of the nurse in the family and community are mentioned but not emphasized in Levine's model. Social utility relates to the model providing clear direction for nursing education, practice, and research. Again the consistent emphasis on the ill, hospitalized individual decreases the social utility except for the hospital environment.

EXTERNAL ANALYSIS OF A MODEL

Nursing Research

Levine places great emphasis on the importance of the scientific method. But use of the scientific method is primarily for the development of hypotheses to guide patient care. Examples of Levine's use of the scientific method are the following:

1. "Nurses may and should use a scientific method in assessment of patient care" (Levine, p 27, 1973).
2. "The scientific method offers the nurse a basis for selecting essential and prior data which will structure the nature of nursing intervention" (Levine, p 28, 1973).
3. "The hypothesis is tested by establishing a protocol of care which will be understood by all persons caring for the patient" (Levine, p 30, 1973).

Research per se is not explicitly stated in Levine's model; but research questions are easily generated from the nine models, for example:

1. Model 2—Body movement and positioning—what effect does bedrest have on the musculoskeletal structure and moods for the hospitalized individual with an orthopedic injury?
2. Model 3—Ministration of personal hygiene needs—what is the effect of the bed, or a bath on body temperature of an elderly ill individual?

Research questions developed from Levine's model would emphasize the ill, hospitalized person.

Nursing Education

Nursing models provide the basis for selecting knowledge to be transmitted in nursing education. Curricula based on theoretical frameworks are necessary if the courses are to form a unified whole. Levine's nursing model was originally written as a textbook for beginning nursing students. Levine attempted to organize scientific principles of bedside care with psychosocial components of the person; this she considered holistic nursing. Levine (1973) states that holistic nursing is dedicated to the humanizing experience that the nurse can bring to the bedside, certain in knowledge and skilled in technique but sensitive and responsive to the patient (p viii). Levine (1973) emphasizes the importance of education by stating that the more the nurse knows, the more likely the nurse will find essential facts provocative, and will develop a testable hypothesis which will provide a valid form of nursing intervention (p 30).

A model of nursing also dictates learning experiences, characteristics of students and faculty, and the educational environment. Levine does not explicitly state an educational environment but does state that her model is to be used in an introductory nursing course. Learning experience for the student would be with ill, hospitalized individuals; patient care would be individualized and structured around the principles of the nursing process.

Nursing Practice

Models of nursing provide a vehicle for awareness of the nature of nursing practice. Levine (1973) states that administratively institutions may vary but if a nurse has nursing knowledge focused on the patient's individualized needs, the nurse can adapt care to fit the setting (p x). Integrated throughout Levine's book are nine models. Each model is a structural framework with scientific concepts and objectives which establish a conceptual pattern so that a wide variety of nursing processes are understood (Levine, p x, 1973).

An example of application of nursing practice from Levine's model would be the care provided Mrs. Smith, who has rheumatoid arthritis. As part of her care, Mrs. Smith takes a warm tub bath every morning. According to Levine, the nurse would know that heat at a specified temperature relieves pain, thus assisting Mrs. Smith's physical movement (conservation of structural integrity). But a bath with warm water too warm would result in body harm. The nurse would provide safety for Mrs. Smith by getting the bath water at the specified temperature as well as assisting her in and out of the tub (conservation of energy). During the bath the nurse would provide privacy and comfort such as proper draping, closing the bathroom door, and providing a tub chair (conservation of personal integrity). Since Mrs. Smith will continue the tub baths at home, the nurse would explain the procedure to her, ask questions about the home environment, and make suggestions regarding the morning bath at home (conservation of social integrity). Throughout the tub bath procedure, the nurse would observe and assess Mrs. Smith in regard to her physical and psychological reaction to the bath, its effect on her motion, her ease at getting in and out of the tub, etc. With the assessment, continuous evaluation and alteration of intervention would occur. Therefore, use of the principle in a model is applicable to a patient situation.

Summary and Evaluation of External Analysis

In evaluating a theory, Hardy (1974) suggests examination of the following: meaning and logical adequacy, operational and empirical adequacy, generalizability, understanding, predictability, and pragmatic adequacy. Applying these evaluatory guides to Levine's model, one must consider Levine's definition of theory. Levine (1966) stated that a theory of nursing must recognize the importance of unique detail of care for a single patient within an empiric framework which successfully describes the requirements of all patients (p 2452). Levine's model has logical adequacy since the unique individual is discussed in regard to nursing practice based on the scientific method. Logical adequacy is diluted by the heavy emphasis Levine places on physical care as compared to psychosocial care of the individual.

Operation and empirical adequacy of a model reflect the model's testability (Hardy, 1974). Levine does not state research questions per se but research questions are readily developed from her model, especially in regard to physical care. Major concepts are adequately defined; and from the concepts, Levine developed nine models which operationally define many terms usable in a research design.

Generalizability of external theory components is restricted due to Levine's great emphasis on the physically ill individual. But the nine models do provide generalizability when providing care to any physically ill individual, thus contributing to the understanding of nursing. Also, Levine's attempt at borrowing knowledge, defining nursing practice, and using the concept of person contributed to the development of nursing science.

The strongest attribute of external analysis in Levine's model is pragmatic adequacy. Since the model was written for beginning nursing students, Levine organized the content in a very pragmatic manner. It ordered nursing education around the concept of the holistic person but the practice setting per se was the hospital.

SUMMARY

Nursing science is a systematic, logical organization of phenomena. Levine (1973) organizes phenomena around the concepts of man, environment, health, and nursing. Man is an ill patient, holistic, dependent, and adaptive. Levine's environment is the hospital; nursing centers around use of the scientific method and the providing of holistic care. Health means whole and encompasses aspects of adaptation. Levine's model has internal and external consistency but is limited in scope to the ill, hospitalized person. Levine altered her model in time to include nursing diagnosis. All in all, Levine's model served as an excellent beginning. Its contribution has added a great deal to the overall development of nursing knowledge.

REFERENCES

Abdellah FG: The nature of a nursing science. Nursing Research, Vol 18, pp 390-393, 1969

Bates M: Naturalist at large. Natural History, Vol 76, p 10, 1967

Dubin R: Theory Building. The Free Press, New York, 1978

Ellis R: Characteristics of significant theories. Nursing Research, Vol 17, No 3, pp 217-222, 1968

Hardy ME: Theories: Components, development, evaluation. Nursing Research, Vol 23, pp 100-107, 1974

Johnson DE: Development of theory: A requisite for nursing as a primary health profession. Nursing Research, Vol 23, pp 371-377, 1974

Levine ME: Adaptation and assessment—a rationale for nursing information. American Journal of Nursing, Vol 66, pp 2450-2453, 1966

Levine ME: The four conservation principles of nursing. Nursing Forum, Vol 6, pp 45-59, 1967

Levine ME: Introduction to Clinical Nursing. F.A. Davis Company, 1969

Levine ME: The intransigent patient. American Journal of Nursing, Vol 70, pp 2106-2111, 1970

Levine ME: Holistic nursing. Nursing Clinics of North America, Vol 6, pp 253-264, 1971

Levine ME: Introduction to Clinical Nursing. F.A. Davis Company, 1973

McKay R: Theories, models, and systems for nursing. Nursing Research, Vol 78, pp 393-400, 1969

Newman MA: Nursing's theoretical evolution. Nursing Outlook, Vol 20, pp 449-453, 1972

Popper KR: Conjectures and Refutations: The Growth of Scientific Knowledge. Harper & Row Publishers, Inc., New York, 1963

Walker LO: Toward a clearer understanding of the concept of nursing theory. Nursing Research, Vol 20, pp 428-435, 1971

8

DOROTHY JOHNSON'S
BEHAVIORAL SYSTEM MODEL

Carol Loveland-Cherry & Sharon A. Wilkerson

INTRODUCTION

Based on Nightingale's contention that nursing's appropriate goal is to assist individuals to prevent or recover from disease or injury, Johnson began to formulate a model for nursing. The development of the model was further influenced by Johnson's knowledge of sociological theory, particularly Talcott Parson's work, and intercultural theories of child-rearing practices. These two bodies of knowledge provided the basis for Johnson's conceptualization of a systems view of the individual in interaction with the environment (Johnson, 1981). Reflected in the development of the model are Johnson's beliefs that nursing as a professional discipline: 1) is not dependent upon medical authority, 2) has a focus different from but complementary to medicine, and 3) has had available a body of relevant facts for nursing care but had not developed a clear theoretical framework or conceptual basis to give direction to the development of the discipline (Johnson, 1961).

BASIC CONSIDERATIONS

In her writings, Johnson has stated that the development of a theory of nursing is not as important as the development of a conceptualization for nursing that "provides direction for practice, education and research" (Johnson, p 2, 1968c). It is towards this end that she proposed a systems model of the individual which serves as the basis for nursing actions and outcomes (Johnson, 1978b). The conceptual model as proposed by Johnson (1968a) would provide a focus for the science of nursing. This model consists of two major components, nursing and person, or man in her terminology. Nursing is identified by its actions and goals and person is described as a behavioral system. The other traditional components of a nursing model, environment and health, are not directly defined, but rather are discussed in terms of their interaction with the behavioral system.

Definition of Nursing

Johnson views nursing as a professional discipline with a distinctive service to offer which encompasses both an art and a science component. A recurrent theme is the necessity to identify and develop the science of nursing based on a common goal. Nursing actions focus on the individual who is attempting to maintain or reestablish equilibrium (Johnson, 1961). Reduction of stress and tension promotes adaptation and stability. Within Johnson's model, nursing is defined as an external regulatory force that assists the individuals to achieve system balance and stability. Therefore, nursing care is based on an understanding of person and his/her responses to change and stress (Johnson, 1959). Johnson (1968b) claims that nursing, as contrasted with medicine, is concerned with the behavioral problems rather than biological functions. However, she emphasizes that nursing problems arise in the area of basic human needs, and the unique area of practice for nursing which is not shared with other health professionals involves such behaviors as feeding, bathing, and toileting (Johnson, 1959).

Nursing Activity

When instability or disequilibrium is evident in the behavioral system, nursing as an external regulator force acts to assist the person to regain stability or equilibrium by either imposing temporary regulatory or control mechanisms or by providing resources to assist the person to meet the functional requirements of the subsystems.

Definition and Understanding of Person

The person (or man in Johnson's terminology) is identified as a behavioral system, which means that he/she is identified by his/her actions and behaviors. These actions and behaviors are regulated and controlled by biological, psychological and sociological factors (Johnson, 1968a, 1968b). As a behavioral system, person is made up of interrelated subsystems. Each of these subsystems affects how individuals will interact with the environment (Johnson, 1974). The actions or behavioral patterns of the total system are efforts to maintain a behavioral system balance while the environmental forces influence the system (Johnson, 1968b). Each person has a unique pattern of actions which distinguishes him/her from other behavioral systems, i.e. other persons. Nursing is concerned with the person as a total entity, which would indicate an involvement with all the subsystems of the behavioral systems.

Definition and Understanding of Health

Health is identified by Johnson (1978a) as an elusive state determined by psychological, social, and physiological factors which is held as a desired value by all the health professions. Based historically on the Nightingale model, the focus of health and illness is the person rather than illness itself. This is contrasted to the medical model which focuses on disease as a biological system disorder (Johnson, 1968a). Health is not seen as a static process, but rather as a moving state of equilibrium which occurs throughout the health change process (Johnson, 1961).

Interrelationship of Components

The interrelationship between person and environment is straightforward in Johnson's model. Environment consists of all factors which are not directly part of the individual behavioral system. These factors act upon the behavioral system which responds in an effort to maintain a balance. The pattern of behavior of an individual determines and limits the interactions between man and environment. Although the main goal of the behavioral system is to achieve a balance, individuals may actively engage in new behaviors that at least temporarily disturb the system balance.

Health problems or lack of balance in the system are either structural or functional. They arise from the system itself or from environmental factors. The five major causes of instability or problems within the system are:

1. Inadequate or inappropriate development of the system or its parts.
2. Breakdown in internal regulatory or control mechanisms.
3. Exposure to noxious influences.
4. Inadequate stimulation of the system.
5. Lack of adequate environmental input (Johnson, 1978b).

Identification of the source of problems in the behavioral system balance leads to appropriate nursing actions. These actions may include:

1. Repairing the structural unit through teaching or similar activities.
2. Temporarily imposing external regulatory or control measures such as limit setting.
3. Providing essential environmental conditions or resources in various situations. An example might be providing contact between mother and infant to facilitate bonding (Johnson, 1978b).

These nursing actions contribute to the achievement of the nursing goal, which is to "maintain or restore a person's behavioral system balance and stability or help a person achieve a more optimal level of functioning (balance) with environmental interactions where possible or desirable" (Johnson, p 2, 1978).

BASIC CONCEPTS

An understanding of system theory is helpful in evaluating Johnson's model of nursing. A system is made up of interrelated subsystems or parts; it is the functioning of these parts together that determines the total system function (Rapoport, 1968). The more complex the system, the greater the number of subsystems that exist in the system. Subsystems are interrelated parts of a system which are linked and open (Johnson, 1980).

Johnson has identified seven subsystems of the behavioral system. These include the attachment/affiliative, the aggressive, the dependency, the achievement, the ingestive, the eliminative, and the sexual systems (Johnson, 1980). The seven subsystems are open, linked, and interrelated. (See Figure 8.3.) Motivational

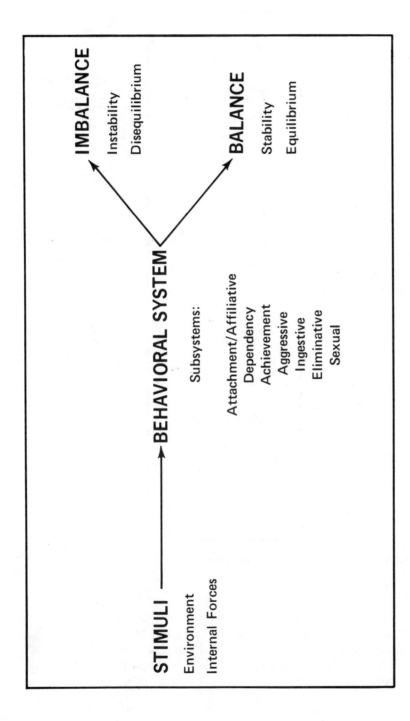

Figure 8.1. Responses of Behavioral System to Stimuli.

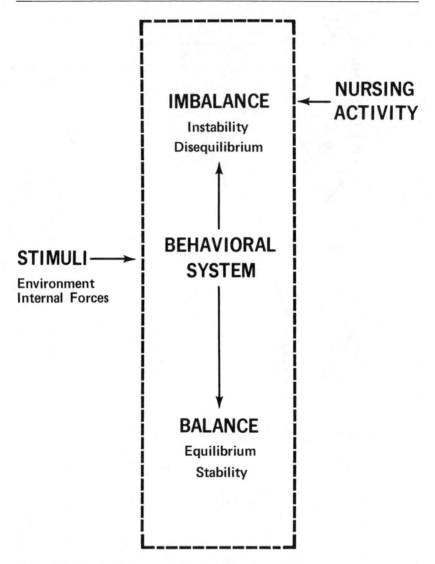

Figure 8.2. Nursing Response to System Imbalance.

drives direct the activities of these subsystems which are continually changing due to maturation, experience, or learning. The
seven subsystems described appear to exist crossculturally and
are controlled by biological, psychological, and sociological factors. Each subsystem can be described and analyzed in terms of
structure, function, and functional requirements. Four structural

elements identified include: 1) drive or goal being sought; 2) set which is the individual's predisposition for a pattern of action; 3) choice which is the group of alternatives for action; and, 4) actions which is the actual behavior of the individual (Johnson, 1980). Each subsystem has the same functional requirements: protection, nurturance, and stimulation. While each subsystem has a specialized function, the system as a whole requires an integrated performance. Therefore, the behavioral system, person, is viewed as a total of the subsystems.

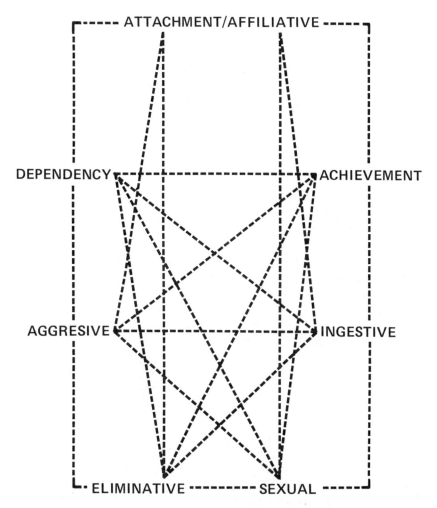

Figure 8.3. Behavioral System: Interrelationships Among Identified Subsystems.

The attachment/affiliative subsystem is identified as the basis of social organization and is proposed to be the first subsystem to emerge developmentally. Security is the general function of this system. Social inclusion, intimacy, and formation and maintenance of a strong social bond are the consequences of the system activities (Johnson, 1980).

The function of the aggressive subsystem is defined as self-protection and preservation. It is recognized that this function exists within the limits of protection and respect of others. Aggression, in this context, is not viewed as a learned, negative response (Johnson, 1980).

The dependency subsystem optimally evolves developmentally from total dependence on others to a large degree of independence with a component of interdependence. Succorance with an expected nurturance response is the general function of the dependency subsystem with consequences of approval, attention or recognition, and physical assistance (Johnson, 1980).

"Mastery or control of some aspect of the self or environment as measured against some standard of excellence" (Johnson, p 213, 1980) is identified as the function of the achievement system. Proposed consequences include physical, creative, mechanical, and social skills.

Behavioral, rather than biological, aspects are the focus of the ingestive and eliminative subsystems. Therefore, appetite satisfaction *per se* is identified as the function of the ingestive subsystem and behavioral excretion of wastes as that of the eliminative subsystem. The emphasis is on when, where, how, what, how much, and under what conditions individuals eat and when, how, and under what conditions individuals eliminate wastes. Social and psychological factors are viewed as not only influencing biological aspects of these systems, but also as, at times, being in conflict with and/or taking precedence over them (Johnson, 1980).

Procreation and gratification are the dual functions of the sexual subsystem. Cultural norms and values as well as biological sex influence the consequences of this subsystem. These consequences include gender identity, courting, and mating (Johnson, 1980).

Other concepts that are necessary for understanding the behavioral system model include equilibrium, stability, instability, stressors and tension. *Equilibrium* is defined as a "stabilized, but more or less transitory, resting state in which the individual is in harmony within himself and with his environment"

(Johnson, p 65, 1961). The system strives for a balance with the external influences, but this does not preclude occasional self-disturbances that result from learning experiences. The adjustments and adaptations in behavior must be useful to the maintenance of the system even if they are not considered to be within the norms for the individual's culture, and all patterns of activity for the system or subsystem serve some purpose (Johnson, 1968b). *Stressors* are stimuli from either internal or external sources, either positive or negative, which impinge upon a system and result in disruption of the stability of the system. *Tension* is defined "as a state of being stretched or strained and can be viewed as a product of disturbance in equilibrium" (Johnson, p 65, 1961). Tension is a potential source of change. Disruption in the structure or function results in a system that needs outside intervention for restoration of balance. Nursing is one such outside intervention force that can help restore the behavioral system to an optimal level.

INTERNAL ANALYSIS

Internal analysis of theoretical models requires examination of both syntax (the logical relationships between units) and semantics (the meaning given to the units) (Hardy, 1974). Therefore, internal analysis of Johnson's model will be conducted along the following areas and criteria:

1. Statement of assumptions
2. Clarity of definitions of units
3. Consistency of use of units and relationships
4. Efficiency of statements of interaction between units
5. Clarity of values inherent in the model and,
6. Adequacy, complexity and scope of model.

Assumptions

Assumptions constitute the foundational core of a theoretical model. Silva (1977) defines these as "statements of general truth that serve as essential premises for whatever is being investigated" (p 61). The assumptions made by Johnson derive from behavioral and systems theory and her philosophical view of nursing. They are consistent with her stated purpose of developing a model to provide direction for nursing practice, education and research. They include:

1. The knowledge required for practice in nursing consists of three types: a) knowledge of order; b) knowledge of disorder; and c) knowledge of control (Johnson, 1968a).
2. ... Nursing is concerned with man as an organized and integrated whole... (Johnson, p 207, 1968a).
3. ... Nursing is concerned with the patient's ability to cope with the situation of illness and with those life situations which might lead to illness (Johnson, p 15, 1968b).
4. Man can be viewed as a behavioral system (Johnson, 1980).
5. ... There is "organization, interaction, interdependency, and integration of the parts and elements" (Chin, 1961) of behavior which makes up the system (Johnson, p 208, 1980).
6. The interrelated parts are called subsystems of behavior (Johnson, 1980).
7. A system "lends to achieve a balance among the various forces operating within and upon it" (Chin, 1961).
8. ... Man strives continually to maintain a behavioral system balance and steady state by more or less automatic adjustments and adaptations to the "natural" forces impinging upon him (Johnson, p 2, 1968c).
9. ... Man also actively seeks new experiences that may disturb his balance, at least temporarily, and that may require small or large behavioral modifications to reestablish balance (Johnson, p 208, 1980).
10. ... A behavioral system, which both requires and results in some degree of regularity and constancy in behavior, is essential to man (Johnson, p 208, 1980).
11. ... Behavioral system balance reflects adjustments and adaptations that are successful in some way and to some degree (Johnson, p 2, 1968c).
12. ... If extraordinarily strong impinging forces, or a lowered resistance to or capacity to adjust to more moderate forces, disturb behavioral system balance, the integrity of the person is threatened (Johnson, p 4, 1968c).
13. ... The attempt by man to preserve, or reestablish behavioral system balance in the face of continuing excessive forces making for imbalance requires an extraordinary expenditure of energy (Johnson, p 4, 1968c).
14. ... Insofar as behavioral system balance requires a minimum (for the moment at least and in reference to a par-

ticular individual) expenditure of energy, a larger supply of energy is available in the service of biological processes and recovery (Johnson, p 4, 1968c).

Central Components

According to Bush (1979), "a model orders, clarifies and systematizes selected components of the phenomena it serves to depict" (p 16). Based on her belief that the patient is the proper focus of nursing action, Johnson presents two major units as basic components of the model: man as a behavioral system and nursing. The behavioral system is a complex unit derived from behavioral and systems theory with the following subunits:

Man: behavioral system

1. Attachment/affiliative
2. Dependency
3. Achievement
4. Aggressive
5. Ingestive
6. Eliminative
7. Sexual

Each subsystem has its own function with consequential behavior, four structural elements—drive, set, choice, action—and the functional requirements of nurturance, protection, and stimulation.

The second major component, nursing, is also a complex unit identified by its goals and actions:

Nursing:

1. Goal—achievement and maintenance of a stable state in behavioral system
2. Actions (three intervention strategies)
   a. Change structural units
   b. Impose temporary external regulatory or control measures
   c. Provide essential environmental conditions or resources.

Definitions

The behavioral system is clearly defined. It is differentiated from the biological system which is identified as the focus of medicine. The subunits of the complex unit, the seven subsystems, are clearly identified and defined in terms of function and structure. The definitions are at an abstract level but have been defined empirically by others (Grubbs, 1980; Holaday, 1980; Rawls, 1980). Empirical indicators are easily extrapolated since the focus is on observable events, actions, or behaviors. For example, empirical indicators of the achievement subsystem could include age appropriate developmental measures such as activities of daily living. Johnson speaks to the necessity of viewing man as a whole. Her definition of person, focused on the totality of the behavioral system, is consistent with this contention. This is efficient since it clearly limits the domain of nursing's concern. It is consistent with Johnson's definition of nursing as a practice discipline focused on the unique aspect of behavior. However, unless the comprehensiveness of Johnson's definition of "behavior" is recognized, confusion may arise regarding the interaction and influence of physiological, psychological and sociological factors.

Johnson defines nursing as an external regulatory force. The goal of nursing is clearly defined and limited. The three intervention strategies identified are consistent with the goal of nursing as defined by Johnson and with the view of man as a behavioral system. The model focuses on the person in potential or actual illness situations, and clearly delineates the concern with the behavioral aspects of illness. While Johnson states that a nursing role exists related to optimizing behavioral system functioning, the nursing actions which are identified focus on individuals who experience either a threat of illness or who are ill. The role of nursing in relation to health maintenance and promotion is not clearly defined. Johnson alludes to the latter two situations in the presentation of her model, but does not develop nor explicate a nursing role.

While both the behavioral system and nursing are major components in Johnson's model, the behavioral system is relegated primary emphasis. This unit is defined in more specific detail and serves as the focal point of the model. Nursing is discussed in terms of the behavioral system, not vice versa. Nursing's goal and actions are predicated upon and defined in terms of the behavioral system. Unless there is instability or less than optimal functioning in the behavioral system, nursing has no identified goal.

Relationships

Dubin (1978) contends that specifying the interactions between units is an indispensable step in developing a scientific model. Johnson's model indicates that the state of the behavioral system determines the type and amount of nursing actions which are necessary. Generally, living systems, including the behavioral system, must maintain both balance and a certain level of stability internally and in interactions with the environment to function efficiently and effectively. Imbalance and/or instability in the system may arise from five sources: 1) inadequate or inappropriate development of the system or its parts; 2) breakdown in internal regulatory or control mechanisms; 3) exposure to noxious influences; 4) inadequate stimulation of the system; or, 5) lack of adequate environmental input (Johnson, 1978b). When a state of imbalance or instability occurs relative to preventing or coping with illness, nursing input is necessitated to maintain or restore equilibrium. This is accomplished via the nursing actions defined in the model. In the latter instance, little information is available regarding the type of role played by the patient. The question can be raised as to whether the relationship between the behavioral system and nursing is interactive or reactive.

The relationships between the two major units can be stated as follows:

> A state of imbalance or instability in the behavioral system results in the need for nursing actions; and appropriate nursing actions results in the maintenance or restoration of behavioral system balance and stability.

Using Dubin's (1978) system of evaluating relationships between units, two sequential laws of interaction are proposed by the model. That is, a state of imbalance or instability must exist before nursing actions are necessary, and appropriate nursing actions must be implemented in order to restore balance and stability in the system. According to Dubin, a sequential law of interaction is one which employs a time dimension to order relationships among units (Dubin, 1978).

Internal Consistency

The units and relationships between units are consistently defined and used except in the instance of the behavioral system being open and having the ability to initiate action. While Johnson implies that the behavioral system is an open, active one in interaction with the environment, the relationships identified between the behavioral system and the environment, including nursing, suggest only that the behavioral system reacts and adapts. Nursing is defined as acting upon the behavioral system; less consideration is evident as to the individual's role in the process of preventing and coping with disturbances or in initiating change or growth. The model does not explicate the potential for active decision making on the part of the individual. Thus, a contradictory situation appears to exist: man is defined as an active, open system but in terms of nursing intervention, becomes, at least temporarily, passive.

The units identified by the model and their definitions are consistent with Johnson's beliefs about the appropriate focus for nursing. The relationships are stated are consistent with the assumptions identified. Additionally, the model consistently reflects Johnson's belief that health is not the sole nor major concern of nursing. The definition of nursing's goal is clearly compatible with an illness model, but less so with a health promotion model. This, however, does not present difficulties in terms of internal consistency; it is a concern in terms of scope, which will be addressed in a later section.

Johnson clearly explicates her value for developing a model for nursing practice, education, and research. The model is consistent with and reflective of this value. The three types of knowledge required for practice in nursing, as identified by Johnson (1968a), are also addressed by the model.

Adequacy

The adequacy of Johnson's model will be addressed using criteria suggested by Ellis (1968), Jacox (1974) and Hardy (1974). Jacox (1974) identifies three levels of theory development: "1) a period of specifying, defining, and classifying the concepts used in describing the phenomena of the field; 2) developing statements or propositions which propose how two or more concepts are related; and 3) specifying how all the propositions are related to each other in a systematic way" (p 5). Johnson's model evidences the criteria for the first two levels. The units of behavioral system and nursing are delimited and defined and statements are developed regarding the relationship between them. The statements of relationship are developed at a general level and are not sufficiently specified or systematized to satisfy the third level of development. However, the model does suggest opportunities for this to be done.

Johnson's definition of nursing in terms of the patient is consistent with Ellis' (1968) contention that "nursing . . . cannot be defined apart from the patient, the definition centers on functions for the patient" (p 218). Scope is a second criterion identified as important to the significance of a theory by Ellis (1968): ". . . (those) most important for nursing would be those that encompass both biological and behavioral observations, and have the potential for explaining their relationships" (p 219). Johnson's model focuses on behavioral aspects but does imply the impact of biological factors. The goal of nursing is clearly defined and delimited. The latter presents some concern in terms of scope. While prevention is incorporated in the definition of nursing's goal, promotion and maintenance are not. Since the emphasis on promotion and maintenance of health as appropriate foci for nursing has evolved subsequent to Johnson's development of the model, inclusion of these concepts cannot be reasonably expected. Also, the model speaks primarily to the individual as the patient. Groups, such as families, are alluded to but not specifically identified as recipients of nursing care. While Johnson does not state that her purpose is to include groups, such as families, this does not preclude this being done in future development of the model. However, some restriction of the types of nursing actions taken and the overall context of the model, i.e. illness-related situations, may provide limited opportunity for further development.

A third characteristic of significant theories is complexity (Ellis, 1968). Either multiple variables and relationships are included or a limited number of variables are viewed in great complexity. The variables in Johnson's model are few and the range of meaning of the variables is somewhat restricted. The behavioral system, however, is treated in detail and complexity with the explication of the subsystems, and their functional and structural properties. The second major unit in the model, nursing, is treated fully. The nursing actions identified reflect the complexity of the behavioral system unit. The syntax of the model is somewhat limited in complexity, dealing primarily with reactive relationships within an illness focus.

Ellis (1968) identifies a fourth criterion of usefulness as an essential characteristic of significant theories for nursing. Theoretical models are not significant if they do not provide guidance for practice. Johnson's behavioral system model clearly provides this guidance in illness-related situations. The role of nursing in non-illness situations is not as clearly defined. However, this can be understood in terms of the era in which the model was first explicated.

In summary, using criteria identified by Ellis (1968), Jacox (1974) and Hardy (1974), the internal analysis of Johnson's model leads to several conclusions. It is a model developed for nursing practice with the two major units—behavioral system and nursing—clearly and consistently defined and used. The scope of the model is largely confined to behavioral aspects of the individual in illness-related situations; this is consistent with Johnson's values and philosophy. It is concluded that Johnson's model is overall clearly defined and meets certain criteria of identifying and defining phenomena and relationships.

EXTERNAL ANALYSIS

Research in nursing has been used to verify conceptual models and has led toward the goals of establishing the scientific base of nursing. Johnson states that nursing in the past was not based upon a scientific foundation, and this situation allows the nurse researcher many choices that are not available to researchers in other fields (1974). It is the nurse researcher who will influence the development of both the scientific discipline and the professional practice of nursing. By choosing one of the nursing models for the basis of research, the researchers not only influence the profession but also determine the direction of their own research. The behavioral system model leads the researcher in two directions. One person might choose to concentrate on the basic sciences, which are investigating the functioning of the subsystems as well as the functioning of the whole behavioral system. Another researcher may choose instead to investigate problems related to the behavioral systems and methods of solving those problems. The area of applied research that deals with identification and solution of problems would be more closely linked to the practice of nursing as identified by Johnson (1959).

Nurse researchers have demonstrated the usefulness of Johnson's model in clinical practice in a variety of ways. The nursing process and assessment has been studied in relation to the behavioral system model (Damus, 1980; Glennin, 1980; Grubbs, 1980; Rawls, 1980). The model has been utilized as a framework for nursing intervention (Damus, 1980; Skolny and Riehl, 1974), and as a model for care of children (Holaday, 1974; Small, 1980). These studies have increased nursing's body of knowledge.

Nursing education based on the behavioral system model would have definite goals, and course planning would be relatively straightforward. A background in biological, psychological, and sociological fields would be necessary for complete understanding of the behavioral system. The main focus of nursing education would be the study of person as a behavioral system. Also included would be the study of behavioral system problems which would require the use of the nursing process in relation to disruptions in the behavioral system functioning. Johnson states that the study of behavioral system problems presents difficulties for curriculum content development because "the knowledge base tends to be disorganized and more intuitive and speculative than scientific" (Johnson, p 215, 1980).

Nursing practice is operationalized by its definition in the behavioral system model. The model itself states the "end product," which is the goal of nursing practice (Johnson, 1968c). Nursing's goal is to maintain or restore the person's behavioral system balance and stability or to help the person achieve a more optimum level of function. Change of any magnitude toward recovery from illness or towards more desirable health practices depends upon the periodic achievement and maintenance, perhaps for only a short time, of this stable state. Thus, with this goal clearly stated, nursing can develop precise measurements for evaluating nursing action effectiveness.

An example of practice based on Johnson's model would be pre-operative teaching. By giving patients information concerning their surgery and what they can expect to have happen both pre-operatively and post-operatively and by providing support by listening to their concerns and questions, their tension, anxiety, and fatigue would be reduced. This reduction would help them to develop attitudes and behaviors that would lead to the achievement of equilibrium. Assessment of the effectiveness of the pre-operative teaching would be included in the nursing process.

SUMMARY

Johnson's model for nursing focuses on the person as a behavioral system which is made up of seven interrelated subsystems. The goal of the behavioral system is to achieve and/or maintain equilibrium. When the behavioral system is in a state of imbalance or instability, nursing activity as an external regulatory force assists the person to regain equilibrium.

The two major components in the model, behavioral system and nursing, are clearly and consistently defined and used. The model as presented emphasizes the individual in a context of threatened or actual illness. Nursing's role in health promotion and maintenance is alluded to but not as clearly developed. Johnson's model provides direction for nursing education, research, and practice.

REFERENCES

Bush HA: Models for nursing. Advances in Nursing Science, Vol 1, pp 13-20, 1979

Chin R: The utility of system models and developmental models for practitioners. In Benne K, Bennis W, Chin R (eds): The Planning of Change, Holt, New York, 1961

Damus K: An application of the Johnson behavioral system model for nursing practice. In Riehl JP, Roy SC (eds): Conceptual Models for Nursing Practice, 2nd ed, Appleton-Century-Crofts, New York, 1980

Dubin R: Theory Building. The Free Press, New York, 1978

Ellis R: Characteristics of significant theories. Nursing Research, Vol 17, No 3, pp 217-222, 1968

Glennin C: Formulation of standards of nursing practice using a nursing model. In Riehl JP, Roy SC (eds): Conceptual Models for Nursing Practice, 2nd ed, Appleton-Century-Crofts, New York, 1980

Grubbs J: An interpretation of the Johnson behavioral system model for nursing practice. In Riehl JP, Roy SC (eds): Conceptual Models for Nursing Practice, 2nd ed, Appleton-Century-Crofts, New York, 1980

Hardy ME: Theories: Components, development, evaluation. Nursing Research, Vol 23, pp 100-106, 1974

Holaday B: Implementing the Johnson model for nursing practice. In Riehl JP, Roy SC (eds): Conceptual Models for Nursing Practice, 2nd ed, Appleton-Century-Crofts, New York, 1980

Jacox A: Theory construction in nursing: An overview. Nursing Research, Vol 23, pp 4-13, 1974

Johnson DE: A philosophy of nursing. Nursing Outlook, Vol 7, pp 198-200, 1959

Johnson DE: The significance of nursing care. American Journal of Nursing, Vol 61, No 11, pp 63-66, 1961

Johnson DE: Theory in nursing: Borrowed and unique. Nursing Research, Vol 17, No 3, pp 206-209, 1968a

Johnson DE: Toward a science of nursing. Southern Medical Bulletin, Vol 56, No 4, pp 13-23, 1968b

Johnson DE: One conceptual model of nursing. Paper presented April 25, 1968c at Vanderbilt University

Johnson DE: Development of theory: A requisite for nursing as a primary health profession. Nursing Research, Vol 23, No 5, pp 372-377, 1974

Johnson DE: State of the art of theory development in nursing. In Theory Development: What, Why, How?, National League for Nursing New York, 1978a

Johnson DE: Behavioral system model for nursing. The 2nd Annual Nurse Educator Conference, 1978b

Johnson DE: The behavioral system model for nursing. In Riehl JP, Roy SC (eds): Conceptual Models for Nursing Practice, 2nd ed, Appleton-Century-Crofts, New York, 1980

Johnson DE: Telephone conversation, October 7, 1981

Rapoport A: Foreword. In Buckley W (ed): Modern Systems Research for the Behavioral Scientist, Aldine, Chicago, Illinois, 1968

Rawls AC: Evaluation of the Johnson behavioral model for clinical practice. Report on a test and evaluation of the Johnson theory, Image, Vol XII, No 1, pp 13-16, 1980

Riehl JP, Roy SC: Conceptual Models for Nursing Practice, 2nd ed. Appleton-Century-Crofts, New York, 1980

Silva MC: Philosophy, science, theory: Interrelationships and implications for nursing research. Image, Vol 9, pp 59-63, 1977

Skolny MA, Riehl JP: Hope: solving patient and family problems by using a theoretical framework. In Riehl JP, Roy SC (eds): Conceptual Models for Nursing Practice, Appleton-Century-Crofts, New York, 1974

Small B: Nursing visually impaired children with Johnson's model as a conceptual framework. In Riehl JP, Roy SC (eds): Conceptual Models for Nursing Practice, 2nd ed, Appleton-Century-Crofts, New York, 1980

9

OREM SELF-CARE MODEL
OF NURSING

Ruth L. Johnston

INTRODUCTION

Dorothea Orem defines nursing as a human service, differentiates it from all other human services, and indicates that nursing's special concern is man's need for the provision and management of self-care action on a continuous basis in order to sustain life and health or to recover from disease or injury (Orem, 1971). Of those who preceded Orem, Henderson's model appears to be the most closely related. Both Henderson and Orem focus primarily on the individual, stress assisting the individual with activities he/she can no longer do for himself/herself, and extend the defined boundaries of nursing to include assisting the individual toward independence from nursing or assistance toward a peaceful death.

Orem first published her model of nursing in 1958. While on the faculty at Catholic University of America she continued her efforts to develop the formalized model of nursing (Orem, 1971, 1980). As a member of the Nursing Development Conference Group, she and others continue to refine her model which she terms a theory for nursing (NDCG, 1973, 1979). Self-care as an organizing model for private practice has been described by Kinlein (1977). The Orem model is being used as a basis for continued curriculum development in several university nursing

137

programs. Orem has been active in the development of a curriculum for the licensed practical nurse, and attends not only to two previously defined levels of nursing, the R.N. and the L.P.N., but also to the associate and baccalaureate degree levels. She identifies the ways in which these levels differ from the first type of educational program, the hospital school of nursing. As additional sources contributing to her conceptualization of nursing, Orem credits Peplau, Orlando, Wiedenbach, and Nagel, whose *Structure of Science* (1961) provided the basis for Orem's approach to a practice theory (Orem, 1980).

BASIC CONSIDERATIONS

Within nursing agreement exists that the concepts of person, environment, health, and nursing are basic to the domain of nursing. Each of these concepts will be defined, followed by definition and discussion of additional concepts central to this model.

Man: Integrated Whole

In discussing the nature of man, Orem reflects man as self-reliant and responsible for self-care and well-being of his/her dependents. Self-care is a requirement for man. It is man's capacity to reflect upon his/her experiencing of himself/herself and his/her environment, and his/her use of symbols (ideas, words) which distinguishes him/her from other species.

Man is viewed as an integrated whole, a unity functioning biologically, symbolically, and socially. The societal influence as a determinant of expectations for man's behavior is strong in the Orem model, and is reflected in the man-environment interaction, but is not clearly defined. Another aspect of unified man limited in this model is the psychological. Orem speaks of needed environmental conditions as either physical or social, and refers to the socializing process as significant. She further discusses internally-oriented behaviors necessary in self-care as those dependent upon awareness, perception, and decision-making as related to self and environment, and upon a state of motivation and interest necessary to learning and applying knowledge. Emotions are mentioned only as something in need of control in order to face the reality of one's health situation.

Environment

Environment as a separate concept is relatively unimportant within this model. Rather, it is a subcomponent of man. Orem elaborates man and environment as an integrated system related to self-care. The existence of environmental factors which have an impact upon the health needs of patients, and thus must be modified by the nurse, is implicit in this model. Further, provision of a developmental environment is offered as a method of assistance. Environmental conditions conducive to development include: opportunities to be helped by being with other persons or groups where care is offered; available opportunities for solitude and companionship; provision of help for personal and group concerns without limiting individual decisions and personal pursuits; shared respect, belief, and trust; recognition and fostering of developmental potential. Each person strives to earn respect and trust as he/she assumes or attempts to assume responsibility for personal development (Orem, 1980).

Health: State of Wholeness

Orem defines health as "state of wholeness or integrity of the individual human being, his parts, and his modes of functioning" (Orem, p 42, 1971). Her definition of health includes the capacity to live as a human being within one's physical, biologic, and social environments and achieve some measure of his/her potential. Just as self-care is used in a variety of ways in this model, so too is the term health. Health is the responsibility of a total society and all of its members. The meeting of health needs requires many health roles and shared or fluctuating responsibilities. The definition of health is to some extent dependent upon one's views of man's human and biologic characteristics and the philosophic view of the discipline to which one belongs. Thus various definitions of health will emerge.

The health-illness continuum with universal self-care and health-deviation self-care defining the ends of the continuum is implied in this model. The components described as self-care demand and self-care limitations also provide a range of health services. Self-care is defined as a deliberate action, the care which all persons require each day. Self-care is an adult's personal, continuous contribution to his/her own health and well-being.

Activities of self-care are learned relative to the beliefs, habits, and practices which characterize the cultural group of the particular individual involved. Much of this is learned in the socializing process of growing up. Conflicts between self-care values and other values may influence the selection of activities to practices which are unhealthy. This too provides the opportunity for a broad range of service. Orem identifies primary, secondary, and tertiary prevention as appropriate to nursing (Orem, 1971, 1980).

Nursing Practice: A Human Service

Nursing provides a human service, arising out of a mandate from society, and like other human services, nursing is a way of overcoming human limitations. It is a personal, family, and community service within the health field, but focuses primarily on the individual, regardless of the context in which it occurs (Orem, 1971, 1980).

Nursing care as viewed by Orem may be continuous or periodic, and has both health and illness dimensions. The main conceptual elements of nursing practice are self-care, including universal self-care and health-deviation self-care, self-care inabilities or limitations, and self-care agency. The goals of nursing practice and the criterion measures of effectiveness are developed around the accomplishment of self-care of a therapeutic quality and around the role of the patient and others in its accomplishment (agency). Agency is defined as "the power of an individual to engage in estimative and production operations essential for self-care" (NDCG, p 118, 1979). The formal object of nursing practice rests with the inabilities of individuals to engage in self-care because of health or health-related reasons. The results are specified in relation to self-care and self-care agency. The results are beneficial to the degree that the patient's self care is accomplished. Nursing actions are helpful in moving the patient toward responsible action in self-care and/or until the family or other non-nurse becomes increasingly competent to provide these actions.

Nursing's special concern or uniqueness rests with the "individual's need for self-care action and the provision and management of it on a continuous basis in order to sustain life and health, recover from disease or injury, and cope with their effects" (Orem, p 6, 1980). The boundaries defined for nursing practice include: it may be required for or by any age group, but it is the situation of health, not the dependencies arising from age which initiates the requirements for nursing; requirements may be modified by progressively favorable change either in the state of health or the increased learning or capacity to be self-directing in self-care. Nursing's relationships in society are based on a state of imbalance between the abilities of nurses to manage and maintain systems of therapeutic self-care for individuals and the abilities of the individuals and their families to provide this. When nurses' abilities are greater, there is a valid need for service; if nurses' and clients' abilities are equal, or the individual's or family's ability is greater, there is no valid basis for nursing service (Orem, 1971, 1980).

Nursing is characterized as action, as assistance. For activities to be considered nursing they must be consciously selected and directed by the nurse toward accomplishing nursing goals. Since nursing functions through a system of activities to meet patient's needs, the system should be designed before any assistance is given. The process of system design is ongoing to provide for needed modification. The nursing system is designed through the selection of methods of assisting which clarify the scope of nursing responsibility, the dimensions of the nursing role, the patient's role, and the reason for the nurse's relationship to the patient.

Orem (1971, 1980) presents three basic nursing systems for organizing nursing services: 1) a wholly compensatory system where acting and doing for the patient is central; 2) a partially compensatory system, where either the nurse or the patient may have the major role; and 3) a supportive-educative system wherein support, guidance, provision of a developmental environment, and teaching are central components. The basic design selected suggests the needed assisting techniques for nursing intervention.

The nursing process guides nursing actions. Nursing process is initiated through assessment in relation to six factors or areas of needed information. These include the patient's health status; the physician's perspective of the patient's health; the patient's perspective of his/her health; the health goals within the context of the patient's life history, life style, and health status; the patient's requirements for therapeutic self-care; and, the patient's capacity to perform therapeutic self-care (Orem, 1971).

Orem further defines nursing situations as including the characteristics of helping situations, methods of assisting which are not unique to nursing and nursing acts. She provides four groups of nursing acts and indicates that learning to nurse and acquiring expertise in nursing involves more than learning how to perform care measures for patients. Orem provides direction to nursing education by delineating the areas of competence which differentiate professional and technical nursing and by indicating knowledge necessary for these competencies.

Nursing acts are specified as belonging to one of the four groups: 1) acts which require judgments as to why patients require nursing; 2) acts which require knowledge of appropriate methods of assisting; 3) acts which result in accomplishment of self-care or overcoming limitations for self-care action; and, 4) acts which result in the adjustment of, or a change in, the system of nursing assistance in order to adapt to presenting conditions and circumstances (Orem, 1971).

Derivation of Nursing: Social Mandate

Nursing arises through a mandate from society which defines the scope, limits and credentials of nursing practice (agency), and the scope and limits of the patient role (patiency). The condition which validates the existence of a requirement for nursing in an adult is the ability to maintain for himself/herself that amount and quality of self-care which is therapeutic. In the child, nursing is validated by the inability of the parent (or guardian) to maintain continuously for the child that amount or quality of self-care which is therapeutic.

Through the nursing process, the nurse selects the nursing model appropriate to the patient, and designs more specifically the system including the nursing situations (helping situations in which patient requirements for care and abilities and assisting acts of the nurse bring about a complementary set of behaviors). The core element of the nursing situation includes what the nurse and patient must do to achieve health goals for the patient. The "person" elements include the patient as a person with all of the contributions of age, sex, physical, intellectual, and emotional manifestations of growth and development, characteristic behaviors, cultural manifestations, and past and present external demands. The nurse as a person includes position factors, the role as agent, and the acceptance of and the willingness to render care. The core elements and person elements combined with the health and disease elements comprise the total.

The Relationships Among Concepts

The concepts of person, nursing practice, and health as described by Orem are interwoven. The major unifying force seems to be defined as society which defines health, mandates agency (at times the responsibility of the adult in the society and at times the responsibility of nursing), spells out clearly under what conditions patiency (receiver of service) is acceptable, and the credentials and scope of the practice of nursing. The broad system—society—thus has a major influence over the man-environment system and the particular nursing selected for the situation. Figure 9.1 shows a graphic illustration.

Relationship of Nursing and Health

Requirements for health maintenance and disease prevention are specified in relation to both human structure and functioning, and to specific diseases or interferences. Effective meeting of universal self-care requisites, considering age, environmental conditions, state of health, and development are the components of health care at the primary level of prevention. Secondary prevention includes prevention of complicating diseases and adverse effects and prolonged disability through early diagnosis and treatment; tertiary prevention focuses on rehabilitation in the event of disfigurement or disability.

The relationship of conditioning factors to health is implicit in this model. The environmental factors conducive to healthy development center around provision of group relationships designed to promote individual growth. Nursing has as its responsibility the provision of a developmental environment when self-care deficits warrant such experiences.

Self-Care: A Many Faceted Concept

The term "self-care" within this model takes on many meanings. As previously defined, self-care is a deliberate action. Additionally, self-care is a requisite for all persons. Orem lists as universal self-care requisites the maintenance of sufficient intake of air, water, and food; provision of care associated with elimination; the maintence of a balance between activity and rest, and between solitude and social interaction; the prevention of hazards to human life, functioning, and well-being; and, the promotion of human functioning and development within social groups in accord with human potential and limitations. Developmental and health care deviation requisites are also categorized (Orem, 1980).

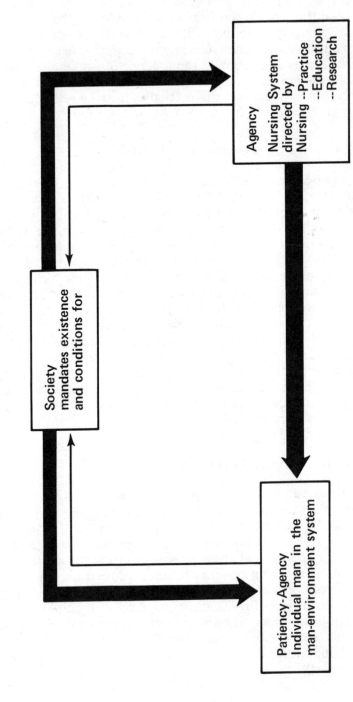

Figure 9.1. Orem Self-Care Model: Interrelationships Among Concepts. (*From*: Fitzpatrick JJ, Whall AL, Johnston RL, Floyd JA: Nursing Models and Their Psychiatric Mental Health Applications. Robert J. Brady Co, Bowie, Maryland, p 59, 1982)

INTERNAL THEORY ANALYSIS

Central Theory Components: Self-Care in Its Many Forms

The central theory components of the Orem model include society, the person as a biologic, symbolizing and social unity, the person-environment system, and self-care in its many forms and conditioning factors. Self-care is defined as the practice of activities that individuals initiate and perform on their own behalf in maintaining life, health, and well-being. Self-care theory, theory of self-care deficits, the theory of systems of nursing, and the nursing process relate these components.

The concept of self-care agency is further elaborated to contain both an operations component and a power component (NDCG, 1979). The operations component includes the ability to perform three types of operations: 1) estimative, or stating what exists; 2) transitional, or deciding what should be done and if it can be done; and 3) productive operations, e.g., doing what needs to be done. The power component includes ten abilities that articulate with the operations component to make up the concept of self-care agency. The power components include the ability to: 1) attend to self as a self-care agent and attend to the internal and external conditions and factors which are significant for self-care; 2) maintain physical energy for initiation and continuation of needed self-care operations; 3) control movements required for initiation and completion of self-care operations; 4) reason within a self-care frame of reference; 5) maintain sufficient motivation; 6) make and operationalize decisions about self-care; 7) acquire, retain, and operationalize technical knowledge for self-care; 8) develop and maintain cognitive, perceptual, manipulative, communicative, and interpersonal skills needed to perform self-care operations; 9) order needed actions into sequential relationships needed for achievement of regulatory goals; and, 10) consistently perform self-care operations within the context of personal, family and community living (NDCG, 1979).

Assumptions of the Orem Self-Care Model

Assumptions underlying self-care, self-care deficits, self-care demand, and self-care capabilities are discussed. The assumptions involving the concept of self-care include: 1) self-care is a requirement of every person; 2) universal self-care involves meeting basic human needs; 3) health-deviation self-care is related to disease or injury; 4) each adult has both the right and the responsibility to care for self in order to maintain rational life and health; she/he may also have responsibilities for dependents; 5) self care is learned behavior processed by the ego and influenced by both self concept and level of maturity; 6) self-care is deliberative action; and, 7) awareness of relevant factors and their meaning is a prerequisite condition for self-care action.

Person-Environment Interaction

Assumptions pertaining to the person-environment interaction include: 1) human functioning is highly integrated at every stage of development; 2) knowledge of anatomic structure, physiologic mechanisms, and unique patterns of response to environmental stimuli are needed to understand integrated human functioning; 3) man's environment forms an integrated whole or system; 4) a highly integrated system can be altered safely only within narrow limits; 5) techniques which persons use to control their environment and functioning are influenced by adaptive forces inherent in man's nature, his/her basic needs and drives, and the creative abilities of the individual and the social groups to which she/he belongs; 6) self-care and dependent care are deliberate actions which involve man-environment interaction; 7) self-care and dependent care are interpreted as inputs into each individual's system of functioning; and, 8) knowledge of the nature of the interchange between individual and environment is basic to introduction of new elements to bring about change.

Agency-Patiency: Social Determinants

In the Orem model, agency may be fully in the domain of nursing responsibility, as with the wholly compensatory system; shared but predominantly the domain of either the nurse or patient in the partly compensatory system; and fully in the hands of the patient in the supportive-educative system with the actions of the nurse geared toward overcoming the patient's self-care limitations. The recipient of service is also delineated in the model, with the conditions under which patiency is accepted, determined by society. Orem is probably the most comprehensive of the theorists in providing the boundaries, specific conditions, learnings, skills, and situations in which nursing may be practiced. She states that the results of nursing are specified in relation to self-care and self-care agency. The results are deemed beneficial to the degree that a) patient's self-care is accomplished, b) nursing actions are helpful in moving the patient toward responsible actions in self-care, or c) the family or other non-nurse becomes increasingly competent (Orem, 1971).

Assumptions on which concepts of agency and patiency are dependent include the social value of self-help and help to others, conditions determined by society for sanctioning agency and patiency, and the self-care focus which validates the existence of nursing.

The procedures, techniques, and protocol for nursing are delineated in the Orem model in: 1) the nursing situations (five are listed, each has characteristics of helping situations); 2) methods of assisting (five general methods, not unique to nursing); 3) assisting techniques, including performing care measures, making appropriate observations and judgments relative to self-care and needs for assistance with it, selecting and securing resources, designing and managing self-care within the patient's system of daily living patterns, initiation, maintenance, and severance of the nurse-patient relationship, socialization of the patient regarding his/her role and the nurse's role, and adaptation and adjustment of the nurse and patient to role changes; 4) the group of nursing acts gives additional direction to the procedure. Specific directions in the use of these to design more fully the nursing system chosen, and the use of the nursing process as the major tool complete the protocol.

Nursing agency is defined as the ability of the nurse to render care. Self-care demand is defined as the unmet need for self-care arising not only from disease, injury, disfigurement, and disability, but also from medical care.

Critique of Consistency and Adequacy

The problems of classifying units of theory in the behavioral sciences necessitates building theories upon selected characteristics or properties of things rather than things themselves. Theory is concerned with modeling the processes and outcomes of particular units interacting in systems. The Orem model demonstrates the process and outcomes of the nursing focus and the processes and outcomes of the basic nursing systems.

In his discussion of attributes and properties, Dubin (1978) differentiates an attribute by the quality of being present; universal self-care and self-care requisites are attributes in the Orem model. A variable is a property of a thing that may be present in degree. The variables in self-care are the health-deviation self-care, the self-care limitations and self-care interferences as well as the self-care conditions and self-care actions taken by either individual or nurse as self-care agents. These then are the major areas for research in this model.

The remainder of assumptions as stated in the Orem model refer predominantly to attributes. However, they contain real units with empirical indicators. The units are for the most part enumerative units.

Other units in the Orem model include the concept of society, which is a summative unit, not clearly defined but all-powerful in its influence over other units of the theory. Man as self-care agent and man having self-care demands are variable units related to health deviation self-care and self-care limitations.

The units of the Orem model relating to nursing practice include the categorizations of types of technologies, groups of diagnoses, nursing situations, groups of nursing acts, methods of assistance, and the nursing process itself. Many of these are associative units, present in some system designs, absent in others. The nursing process may be viewed as an enumerative unit containing its own specific laws of interaction. The three nursing systems draw from the previously named associative units, with clearly defined boundaries and laws of interaction. The units discussed in the man-environment system are also laws of interaction.

The propositions of this model are formulated as a system of nursing is designed. They are formulated in the nursing assessment process, predict outcomes, select situations in which those outcomes may be achieved, select methods of assistance, and needed technologies to design the nursing acts (self-care actions) necessary to achieve these outcomes. The boundaries are clearly established by the system selection and design.

From the study of the Orem model by the Dubin criteria, one would conclude that this model was developed primarily through the inductive process, drawn from extensive experience in nursing practice within a somewhat implicit deductive frame of reference. The deductive components seem to arise from the Thomasian view of man. Society is not specifically defined but seems to have strong predetermined implications from this view. Man as a rational, responsible being with high value placed on self-reliance and responsibility for others is compatible with this view. There are relatively few summative units in this model. This writer believes the model largely fulfills the Dubin requirements of theory building and has the potential to generate many testable hypotheses for nursing interventions. Orem offers descriptive data, based on research to increase understanding and set the stage for prediction in each designed system of nursing. Although the degree of specificity limits the domain and thus the generalizability, the systems, clearly defined, still have considerable breadth while guiding and controlling the practice of nursing. Viewing theory from the degree of abstractness, and compatible with the more inductive emphasis, Orem's theory of nursing seems to be predominantly middle range.

EXTERNAL THEORY ANALYSIS

Operational Mode Inherent in Orem Theory

Orem (1980) views her theory as a technological system modeled after action theory as defined by Nagel (1961). It assumes the existence of contractual and interpersonal systems. The methodology or operational mode of this theory involves the nursing process, initiated through assessment of the universal properties as well as health deviation characteristics as viewed by patient, nurse, and doctor. To do this the nurse must also evaluate the structural and functional wholeness of the patient and his/her life style patterns. The social transaction of the nurse-patient relationship is described as an I—you relationship.

Research Upon the Self-Care Model

As was previously mentioned, the research thrust of this theory is in the area of increasingly effective nursing actions to meet self-care demands. The situations are sufficiently well-defined to generate hypotheses and anticipate empirical indicators in the area of study. It is limited in relation to broader knowledge concerns.

Research which has been conducted upon this model is relatively extensive, focusing on aspects of nursing practice (Backscheider, 1974; Clinton, et al., 1977; Kinlein, 1977a, 1978; Pridham, 1971), nursing education (Piemme and Trainor, 1977), and supervision and administration of nursing services (Anna, et al., 1978; Allison, 1973; Backscheider, 1971). Instrument development is also underway. Among instruments to measure self-care agency are the Performance Test of Activities of Daily Living

(PADL) developed and tested by Kuriansky, Gurland, Fleiss, and Cowan (1976), the measure of the Exercise of Self-Care Agency by Kearney and Fleischer (1979), and an instrument developed by Denyes (1981) to measure self-care agency in adolescents. The Kearney et al. tool is unclear in its conceptualization of "exercise of self-care agency." Since self-care agency is defined as the power of an individual to engage in estimative and productive operations essential for self-care, and is broadened to include the components identified by Kearney and Fleischer. It would seem that a measure of "self-care agency" rather than a measure of the exercise of self-care agency would be more useful in testing this portion of Orem's model. Exercise of self-care agency might more appropriately be based on observed behaviors rather than a mix of capabilities and self-report of activities either in retrospect or prospect.

Education for Self-Care Nursing

This model gives considerable direction to nursing education, delineating many of the skills, techniques, and methods which must be learned to become a practitioner. Orem further defines the relationships which are appropriate, the basic systems within which the nurse practices and thus must learn, and in defining the groups of nursing acts which the nurse must learn to do, and the groups of nursing diagnoses with which she must deal in order to select and design appropriate self-care actions within the appropriate nursing system. She emphasizes that the four groups of nursing acts indicate a level of learning required which is greater than learning to perform care measures for patients. The aspects of nursing discussed in nursing practice, and the learning of interpersonal relationships including communication, teaching, attitude change necessary to an acceptance, and willingness to render care must be a part of the education of the nurse. Further, nurses need to know the conditions and constraints of society on nursing practice, including a comprehensive awareness of the relationship of the nurse and the law.

There are some indications in the discussion of the education and skill of the professional nurse which may be indicative of greater flexibility in the model than is explicitly stated. This is interpreted from the stated expectation that the professional designs systems where the known techniques are not adequate, while the technical nurse operates within systems where techniques are established. Perhaps further study would expose additional areas open to expansion and further development. Indeed, Orem continues to develop the model, and presents changes in emphasis not yet fully explored in either her own book, or the NDCG publications.

The Self-Care Model of Nursing Practice

The major focus of this model is nursing practice. The "proper object" of nursing practice is the individual in a variety of contexts. Orem extends the guidelines for nursing practice to include skilled observation not only of the patient but also of the other elements of the nursing situation: 1) designing the system of nursing for the patient to include delegation of responsibility for some aspects of care to another nurse; 2) supervising and evaluating those functions; 3) redesigning the system as needed; and 4) communicating and coordinating to insure effectiveness. The latter requires relating and teaching others to relate.

Orem delineates the professional and technical levels of nursing practice. For the professionally educated nurse, emphasis is upon the intellectual aspect of the art of nursing so that she can learn to function effectively in nursing situations where the patient's requirements are complex and sometimes obscure, and where techniques for assisting are not well developed. The technical level develops the intellectual aspect in relation to nursing situations where selected assisting techniques and techniques of health care are known to have a high degree of effectiveness (Orem, 1971).

The model seems to have medical overtones in the practice situations. For example, in her discussion of the parts of the nursing focus, Orem (p 128, 1980) lists six components, the first being the physician's perspective of the patient's health situation. Further, in discussing "health care" in relation to prevention, Orem is frequently referring to illness care, delineating methods of nursing care in relation to medically prescribed or endorsed measures of diagnosis, treatment, and rehabilitation. Even when regrouping nursing situations by "health focus," Orem describes "recovery" as a major group, and identifies medical evaluation, medical therapy, medical diagnosis of complications with prompt treatment, etc. For a second major group, "illness of undetermined origin," Orem indicates that health care is organized around signs and symptoms, degree of illness, and need for medical diagnosis. The fifth health focus, regulation through active treatment of a disease, disorder or injury of determined origin follows this same pattern (Orem, 1980). However, Kinlein (1977a) reported that the self-care model is effective as a basis for independent nursing practice. The medical influence may be more a problem of the examples used than an inherent component.

Critique of the External Consistency of the Model

Nursing is a human service to populations who can be helped through nursing. These include those with deficit relationships between current or projected self-care capability and the qualitative or quantitative demand for care.

Nursing activities are summarized under five areas: 1) entering into and maintaining relationships; 2) determining how and if patients can be helped through nursing; 3) responding to patients' requests, desires, and needs for contacts and assistance; 4) prescribing, providing, and regulating direct help in the form of nursing services; and 5) coordinating and integrating nursing with patients' daily living, other health care, and social and educational services.

Orem classifies nursing situations into seven groups: 1) circumstances in relation to the life cycle; 2) those oriented to the process of recovery; 3) those oriented to illnesses or disorder of undetermined origin; 4) those related to genetic or developmental defects; 5) regulation through active treatment of disease, disorder, or injury of determined origin; 6) those situations in which the health focus is oriented to the restoration, stabilization, or regulation of integrated functioning, and, 7) the regulation of serious disruptions to human integrative functions.

SUMMARY

Orem provides a high degree of specificity and seems to include all major aspects of theory in her model. However, because of the specificity to given situations, many groupings, lists, and systems are needed. Thus, the model is not organized in a simple fashion. There are some problems with overlapping and some awkwardness in terminology. However, once the various uses of terminology (e.g. self-care actions, self-care demand, self-care agency shared with others) are mastered, the directions for nursing practice, education, and research become clear.

Orem discusses her theories relevant to the nursing focus as the index or key in estimating the complexity of the nursing situation and thus determining the kinds or levels of nursing preparation needed to meet the patient's requirement. She discusses necessary knowledge and motivation, person elements of both patient and nurse and the availability of resources as she considers the health service or community service needed and the professional service, organization, and influence impinging upon the practitioner.

This model has the potential for generating many hypotheses and in fact has done so. It was designed more to guide practice than to provide a body of substantive knowledge. In this regard the model seems reasonably complete. Although greater emphasis on the nature of man which could broaden the perspective of nursing might be preferred, the values of the theory are implicit. There is, however, a lack of parsimony.

Ellis (1968) looks at scope, complexity, and testability as criteria for evaluating theories. The scope within the theory for guiding practice provides a necessary framework for ordering observations about a variety of phenomena within this context. Again the complexity is such to include multiple variables and attributes and the relationships involved. As to testability, which Ellis discusses as a needed tentativeness to provide flexibility, the implied values in the Orem model seem rather absolutist, limiting the tentative nature, and thus perhaps limiting the flexibility of the model.

Hardy (1974) considers pragmatic adequacy as an important criterion. Orem's model does demonstrate the ability to control the phenomena of interest, the self-care demands, and the self-care actions designed to meet them. The specificity provides a high degree of usefulness in the current practice situation, but is more limited in creating alternatives. Overall, the theory demonstrates a relatively high degree of internal consistency and pragmatic adequacy for nursing practice.

There is a preponderance of inductive elements in this model, which are evident as one views the development of the basic concepts. Throughout her writings, Orem has presented a view of nursing as an applied science and an art.

REFERENCES

Allison SE: A framework for nursing action in a nurse-conducted diabetic management clinic. Journal of Nursing Administration, pp 53-60, July-August, 1973

Anna D, Christensen D, Hohon S, Ord L, Wells S: Implementing Orem's conceptual framework. Journal of Nursing Administration, Vol 8, pp 8-11, 1978

Backscheider J: The use of self as the essence of clinical supervision in ambulatory patient care. Nursing Clinics of North America, Vol 6, pp 785-794, 1971

Backscheider J: Self-care requirements, self-care capabilities, and nursing systems in the diabetic nurse management clinic. American Journal of Public Health, Vol 64, pp 1138-1146, 1974

Clinton J, Denyes M, Goodwin J, Koto E: Developing criterion measures of nursing care: Case study of a process. Journal of Nursing Administration, Vol 7, pp 41-45, 1977

Denyes, MJ: Measurement of self-care agency in adolescents. Presented at ANA Council of Nurse Researchers Annual Conference, Washington, D.C., September, 1981

Dubin R: Theory Building. The Free Press, New York, 1978

Ellis R: Characteristics of significant theories. Nursing Research, Vol 17, No 3, pp 217-222, 1968

Hardy ME: Theories: Components, development, evaluation. Nursing Research, Vol 23, No 2, pp 187-188, 1974

Kearney B, Fleishcher B: Development of an instrument to measure exercise of self-care agency. Research in Nursing and Health, Vol 1, p 25, 1979

Kinlein ML: The self-care concept. American Journal of Nursing, Vol 77, pp 598-601, 1977a

Kinlein ML: Independent Nursing Practice with Clients. J.B. Lippincott, Co., Philadelphia, Pennsylvania, 1977b

Kinlein ML: Point of view on the front: Nursing and family and community health. Family and Child Health, pp 57-68, 1978

Kuriansky J, Gurland B, Fleiss J, Cowan D: The assessment of self-care capacity in geriatric psychiatric patients by objective and subjective methods. Journal of Clinical Psychology, Vol 32, pp 95-102, 1976

Nagel E: Structure of science. Harcourt, Brace and World, New York, 1961

Nursing Development Conference Group: Concept Formalization in Nursing: Process and Product. Little, Brown & Co., Boston, Massachusetts, 1973

Nursing Development Conference Group. Concept Formalization in Nursing: Process and Product, 2nd ed. Little, Brown & Co., Boston, Massachusetts, 1979

Orem DE: Nursing: Concepts of Practice. McGraw-Hill Co., New York, 1971

Orem DE: Nursing: Concepts of practice, 2nd ed. McGraw-Hill Co., New York, 1980

Piemme JA, Trainor MA: A first-year nursing course in a baccalaureate program. Nursing Outlook, Vol 25, pp 184-187, 1977

Pridham KF: Instruction of a school-age child with chronic illness for increased responsibility in self-care, using diabetes mellitus as an example. International Journal of Nursing Studies, Vol 8, pp 237-246, 1971

Riehl JP, Roy C: Conceptual Models for Nursing Practice. Appleton-Century-Crofts, New York, 1974

Riehl JP, Roy C: Conceptual Models for Nursing Practice, 2nd ed. Appleton-Century-Crofts, 1980

Silva M: Selection of a theoretical framework. In Krampitz S, Pavlovich N: Readings for Nursing Research, C.V. Mosby Co., St. Louis, Missouri, pp 17-28, 1981

10

THE ROY ADAPTATION MODEL

Mary E. Tiedeman

INTRODUCTION

Roy (1976b, 1980) began her work on the Adaptation Model of Nursing in 1964 when she was a graduate student at the University of California, Los Angeles. In a seminar with Dorothy E. Johnson, Roy was challenged to develop a conceptual model for nursing. The concept of adaptation impressed Roy as a conceptual framework appropriate for nursing. The work on adaptation by Helson (1964), a physiologic psychologist, was added to the beginning concept and in subsequent years the model was developed as a framework for nursing practice, research, and education. According to Roy (1980), the use of the model in nursing practice led to further clarification and refinement of the model. A pilot research study in 1971 and a survey research study in 1976-1977 led to some tentative confirmations of the model.

As Roy has continued to clarify and refine the model, she has drawn upon the works of other experts in the area of adaptation. The model, as currently explicated, draws upon the works of Dohrenwend (1961), Lazarus (1966), Mechanic (1970), and Selye (1978), as well as the work of Helson (1964).

BASIC CONSIDERATIONS
INCLUDED IN THE MODEL

Roy identifies three essential elements in her model of nursing: 1) the recipient of nursing; 2) the goal of nursing; and, 3) nursing intervention (Roy, 1976b; Roy and Roberts, 1981). These essential elements include the concepts of nursing, person, health-illness, environment, and adaptation.

Definitions of Nursing-Person-Health-Environment

Roy (1976b) defines nursing as "a theoretical system of knowledge which prescribes a process of analysis and action related to the care of the ill or potentially ill person" (p 3). Adaptation nursing is further defined as "an approach to nursing which views man as a biopsychosocial being with modes of adapting to a changing environment, and which acts through a nursing process to promote man's adaptation in each of these modes in situations of health and illness" (p 3). Adaptation nursing consists of both the goal of nursing and nursing intervention (Roy, 1976b; Roy and Roberts, 1981).

According to Roy (1976b), the person "is a biopsychosocial being in constant interaction with a changing environment" (p 11). In her more recent works, Roy describes the person as an adaptive system (Roy, 1980; Roy and McLeod, 1981; Roy and Roberts, 1981).

Roy (1976b) defines the health-illness continuum as "a continuous line representing states of degrees of health or illness that a person might experience at a given time" (p 4). Health-illness is considered by Roy (1970, 1971, 1976b, 1980) to be an inevitable dimension of the person's life.

Environment is defined by a dictionary definition. Environment is "all conditions, circumstances, and influences surrounding and affecting the development of an organism or group of organisms" (Roy and Roberts, p 43, 1981). According to Roy, additional theoretical work on the model is necessary to further clarify environment as distinct from internal stimuli (Roy and Roberts, 1981).

Description of Nursing Activity (Nursing Process)

Nursing is concerned with the person as a total being, interacting with a changing environment and responding to stimuli present because of his/her position on the health-illness continuum (Roy, 1970, 1971, 1973, 1980). When unusual stressors or weakened coping mechanisms make a person's usual attempts to

Table 10.1

Definition of Terms as Used in the Roy Adaptation Model

Adaptive responses	are "those that promote the integrity of the person in terms of the goals of survival, growth, reproduction, and self-mastery" (Roy and Roberts, p 43, 1981).
Ineffective responses	are those which disrupt the integrity of the person and do not contribute to the goals of survival, growth, reproduction, and self-mastery (Roy, 1976b; Roy and Roberts, 1981).
Stress	is "the general term given to the transaction between environmental demands for adaptation and the person's response (Roy and McLeod, p 56, 1981).
Coping	"refers to the routine, accustomed patterns of behavior to deal with daily situations as well as to the production of new ways of behaving when drastic changes defy the familiar responses" (Roy and McLeod, p 56, 1981).
Needs	are requirements within the person which stimulate a response to maintain integrity (Roy, 1976b, 1976d, 1980).
Adaptation problems	are "the occurrences of situations of inadequate response to need deficits or excesses" (Roy, p 4, 1976b).
Focal stimuli	are the stimuli immediately confronting the person (Roy, 1970, 1976b; Roy and Roberts, 1981).
Contextual stimuli	are all other stimuli which are present (Roy, 1970, 1976b; Roy and Roberts, 1981).
Residual stimuli	are factors from past experiences which may be relevant to the present situation but whose current effect cannot be validated. These factors include beliefs and attitudes (Roy, 1970, 1976b; Roy and Roberts, 1981).

ffective, then, the person needs a nurse (Roy and Roberts,

Nursing consists of both the goal of nursing and nursing intervention. The goal of nursing is to promote adaptation of the client in regard to the four adaptive modes: 1) physiologic needs; 2) self-concept; 3) role function; and 4) interdependence. The goal of nursing is reached when the focal stimulus is within the zone set up by the client's adaptation level, i.e., when the focal stimulus falls within a range where the client is able to make an adaptive or effective response. Adaptation frees the client to respond to other stimuli, thus leading to the intended consequences of the model—higher level wellness (Roy, 1970, 1973, 1976b, 1980; Roy and Roberts, 1981).

The goal of adaptation is fostered by the process of assessment and intervention (Roy, 1970). "The adaptation model determines what data to collect, how to identify the problem, what approach to use and how to evaluate the approach" (Roy, p 23, 1976b). The units of analysis of nursing assessment are the person in interaction with his/her environment. The mode of nursing intervention is manipulation of parts of the system or the environment (Roy, 1980).

The assessment process involves two levels of assessment. The first level of assessment is the collection of data relevant to the four modes, i.e., the nurse gathers data about the client's behaviors in each of the adaptive modes. This means that through observation, measurement of responses, and communication with the client the nurse gathers data about each of the adaptive modes: physiologic needs, self-concept, role function, and interdependence. From these data the nurse makes a tentative judgment about whether behaviors are adaptive or ineffective. The second level of assessment is the collection of data regarding focal, contextual, and residual stimuli. During this level of assessment the nurse identifies the factors that influence the behaviors observed in the first level of assessment. The result of the overall assessment is nursing diagnoses which identify the source of difficulty, i.e., need deficits or excesses which lead to ineffective behavior (Roy, 1971, 1976b, 1980; Roy and Roberts, 1981).

Nursing intervention is carried out within the context of the nursing process and involves manipulating the focal, contextual, and residual stimuli so that the stimuli will fall within the zone set up by the patient's adaptive level. This manipulation may involve increasing, decreasing, or maintaining stimulation. Manipulation of focal stimuli may cause them to fall within the zone set up by the patient's adaptation level; whereas manipulation of contextual and residual stimuli may broaden this zone (Roy, 1976b, 1980; Roy and Roberts, 1981).

Thus, it can be seen that nursing intervention includes both a focus and a mode. The focus is adaptation problems, while the mode is changing stimuli through the process of assessment, diagnosing, planning, effecting, and evaluating nursing care (Roy, 1980). Within the model the patient is respected as an active participant in his/her care. Goal setting is mutually agreed upon and manipulation of stimuli is not manipulation of the person (Roy, 1976d; Roy and Roberts, 1981).

Understanding of Person

Roy describes the person as a biopsychosocial being and a living, adaptive* system. In Roy's recent works the emphasis has been on the person as an adaptive system. As a system the person can be described in terms of input, internal and feedback processes, and output. The person receives input externally from the environment and from the self. The output of the system is adaptive and ineffective responses. Through feedback processes these responses provide further input for the person as a system (Roy and McLeod, 1981; Roy and Roberts, 1981).

As a living system the person is an open system and exchanges energy and matter with the environment. The person as a living, open system is negentropic and subject to internal and external stress (Roy and McLeod, 1981; Roy and Roberts, 1981).

The person as a living system is "a whole made up of parts or subsystems that function as a unity for some purpose" (Roy and McLeod, p 53, 1981). Roy has identified six major subsystems of the person (see Table 10.1). These subsystems are two major internal processor mechanisms—the regulator and the cognator—and four adaptive modes—physiologic needs, self-concept, role function, and interdependence (Roy, 1970, 1971, 1976b, 1976d, 1980; Roy and McLeod, 1981; Roy and Roberts, 1981).

These regulator and cognator subsystems are primary; as such they are the mechanisms of adapting or coping with a changing environment. Coping mechanisms are both innate and acquired, i.e., some mechanisms are genetically determined or are

---

*Concepts specific to adaptation will be discussed later in the chapter.

common to the species while other mechanisms are acquired through processes such as learning. The regulator and cognator mechanisms are viewed by Roy as biologic, psychologic, and social in origin, and as methods or ways of coping. She has proposed that they act in relation to the four adaptive modes: physiologic needs, self-concept, role function, and interdependence (Roy, 1970, 1976b, 1980; Roy and McLeod, 1981; Roy and Roberts, 1981).

Table 10.2

Subsystems of the Person as an Adaptive System

Primary/Functional Subsystems (Mechanisms)	Secondary/Effector Subsystems (Modes)
Regulator	Physiologic Needs
Cognator	Self-concept
	Role Function
	Interdependence

The four adaptive modes are seen by Roy as secondary or effector subsystems, i.e., the modes provide the particular form or manifestation of cognator and regulator activity. Therefore, they are more effectors of adaptation than means of adaptation. Behind each of the four modes is a basic need for integrity. This basic need for integrity includes physiologic, psychic, and social integrity (Roy, 1976b; Roy and McLeod, 1981; Roy and Roberts, 1981).

Thus, according to Roy "the person utilizes cognator and regulator mechanisms to adapt to the changing environment. Cognator and regulator activity is effected through the four adaptive modes" (Roy and Roberts, p 71, 1981). This relationship can be seen in Figure 10.1.

With the exception of the physiologic needs mode, Roy describes each of the six subsystems of the person in terms of systems characteristics, i.e., input, internal and feedback processes, parts or subsystems, and output. The relationships among the six major subsystems of the person will be briefly examined.

Roy has identified the processes of the regulator and cognator in a series of propositions.* These processes link together

---

*Propositions related to all subsystems are found in Roy C, Roberts SL (eds): Theory construction in nursing: An adaptation model. Prentice-Hall, Inc., Englewood Cliffs, New Jersey, 1981.

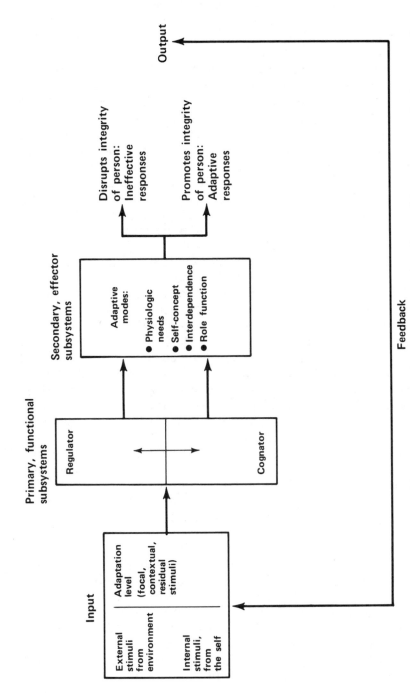

Figure 10.1. The Person: A Living, Adaptive System. (Adapted from Roy C, McLeod D: Theory of the person as an adaptive system. *In* Roy C, Roberts SL (eds): Theory Construction in Nursing: An Adaptation Model. Prentice-Hall, Inc., Englewood Cliffs, New Jersey, p 58, 1981)

the four adaptive modes of physiologic needs, self-concept, role function, and interdependence. According to Roy, the regulator is related predominantly to the physiologic needs mode. The propositions of the regulator are applied to each of the physiologic needs and are related to adaptive and ineffective responses.

Roy views the cognator as related to each adaptive mode in at least three ways. First, each mode provides specific relevant input for the cognator, e.g., feelings of adequacy with regard to self-concept are an important factor in considering emotion and defenses to seek relief. Second, the adaptive mode under consideration will specify the relevant pathways and apparatus, e.g., the learning apparatus seems particularly relevant to the role function mode. Third, within each mode it is possible to view specific cognator processes, e.g., a cognator process that is active in relation to the self-concept is the process of defenses to seek relief (Roy and McLeod, 1981).

The process of perception is found in both the regulator and cognator; it is viewed by Roy as the process which links these two subsystems. "Inputs to the regulator are transformed into perception. Perception is a process of the cognator. The responses following perception are feedback into both the cognator and the regulator" (Roy and McLeod, p 67, 1981). Thus, Roy views the relationship between the regulator and cognator as a hierarchical relationship (Roy and McLeod, 1981). For example, the person receives neural input to the regulator regarding a decrease in environmental temperature. This is transformed into a conscious perception of being cold. This perception is a function of both the regulator and the cognator. Output or responses from the regulator, e.g., shivering, and the cognator, e.g., decision to put on a sweater, are feedback into both the regulator and the cognator. These outputs from the regulator and the cognator are effected through the adaptive modes. For example, shivering is expressed or effected through the physiologic needs mode.

Roy identifies sets of propositions related to the subsystems of the self-concept, role function, and interdependence modes. These propositions relate and link together the parts of each subsystem (Roy and Roberts, 1981). In addition the following relationships can be observed among the four modes. First, internal and external changes may affect more than one adaptive mode simultaneously, e.g., the loss of a leg in an accident would affect physiologic needs, self-concept, and role function. Second, one behavior may be a manifestation of disruption in more than one mode, e.g., loss of weight could involve nutritional deficits or self-concept deficits. Finally, each adaptive mode may act as a focal, contextual, or residual stimulus for each of the other modes. For example, as a child develops his/her role as a student, one of the primary residual factors influencing the situation is how he/she feels about himself/herself—his/her self-concept (Roy, 1971, 1976b).

Thus, the integrated nature of the person as an adaptive system may be seen by the relationships between the regulator and cognator and the adaptive modes. An abstract view of these relationships is demonstrated in Figure 10.2.

Understanding of Health

There is little discussion of the concept of health within the model. Roy (1976b) defines health-illness as a continuum ranging from peak wellness to death with varying degrees of health or wellness in between these extremes. Roy (1970, 1971, 1976b, 1980) views health-illness as an inevitable dimension of the person's life; it is this dimension with which nursing is concerned.

Roy specifies a number of interrelationships among the concepts of person, environment, health, and nursing. The person, a biopsychosocial being and an adaptive system, is in constant interaction with a changing environment. The person as an open system exchanges matter and energy with the environment. Health-illness is viewed by Roy as an inevitable dimension of the person's life. The person receives stimuli from the environment in the dimensions of his/her life related to health and illness.

Nursing is concerned with the person as a total being interacting with the environment and responding to stimuli present because of his/her position on the health-illness continuum. Roy states that nursing is needed when unusual stressors or weakened coping mechanisms make the person's usual attempts to cope ineffective (Roy, 1970, 1971, 1973, 1976b, 1980; Roy and McLeod, 1981; Roy and Roberts, 1981).

Adaptation is a central component in Roy's model of nursing. In viewing man as an adaptive system, adaptation is considered to be both the process of coping with stressors and the end product of coping. The process of adaptation includes all the person's interactions with the environment and is a two-part process. The first part of the process is initiated by changes in the internal or external environment which lead to need deficits or excesses.

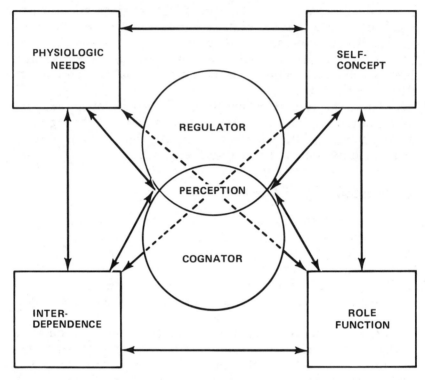

Note: There is direct interaction between all of the adaptive modes and
    between each adaptive mode and the regulator and the cognator.

Figure 10.2. Relationships Among the Subsystems of the Person. (Adapted from
Abstract view of the primary and secondary systems of the Roy Adaptation Model.
In Roy C, Roberts SL (eds): Theory Construction in Nursing: An Adaptation
Model. Prentice-Hall, Inc., Englewood Cliffs, New Jersey, p 186, 1981)

These changes which demand a response are stressors, or focal
stimuli, and are mediated by contextual or residual factors. These
stressors partially produce the interaction called stress. The
second part of the process is the coping mechanisms which are
triggered off to produce adaptive or ineffective responses (Roy,
1980; Roy and McLeod, 1981). This process of stress adaptation is
shown in Figure 10.3.

   The product of adaptation is a result of the process of
adaptation and may be described in terms of conditions that
promote the goals of the person including survival, growth,
reproduction, and mastery. This end state is a state of dynamic

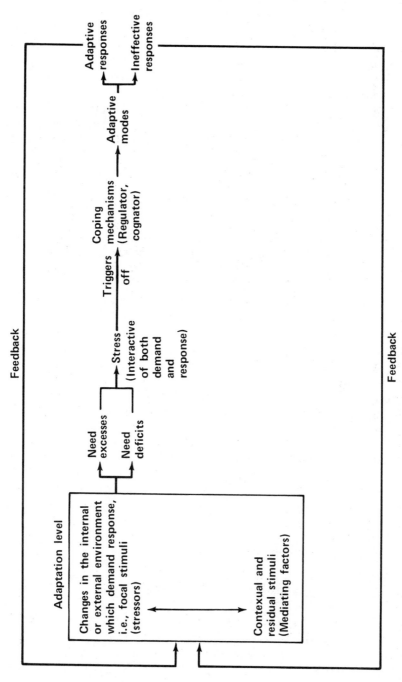

Figure 10.3. The Process of Stress Adaptation. (Adapted from Roy C, McLeod D: Theory of the person as an adaptive system. *In* Roy C, Roberts SL (eds): Theory Construction in Nursing: An Adaptation Model. Prentice-Hall, Inc., Englewood Cliffs, New Jersey, p 54, 1981)

equilibrium which involves both heightened and lowered responses. Each "new adaptive state has affected the adaptation level so that the dynamic equilibrium of the person is at an ever higher level. Greater ranges of stimuli can be dealt with successfully by the person as an adaptive system" (Roy and McLeod, p 60, 1981), thus, promoting adaptation leads to higher level wellness (Roy and McLeod, 1981; Roy and Roberts, 1981).

An important concept with regard to adaptation is that of adaptation level. The adaptation level is the condition of the person relative to adaptation. The adaptation level is the pooled effect of focal, contextual, and residual stimuli and is a variable standard against which feedback can be compared. This constantly changing level (point) represents the person's own standard range of stimuli that he/she will tolerate with ordinary adaptive responses. This range within which stimuli will elicit positive responses is set up by the adaptation level and is known as the adaptive zone. Stimuli that hit outside the zone will elicit a negative response (Roy, 1970, 1976b, 1980; Roy and McLeod, 1981; Roy and Roberts, 1981).

Adaptation, then, is a function of the stimuli coming in and the adaptation level. More specifically it is a function of the gradient between focal stimulus and adaptation level. An adaptive response may occur in two ways. The gradient may be such that the stimulus is within the adaptation zone and the usual responses are adequate. For example, the person who has been immunized against the flu is exposed to the influenza virus. This stimuli would be within his/her adaptive zone and the usual responses would be adequate. Secondly, if the gradient is steeper, i.e., the stimulus is outside the adaptation zone, then "initial efforts to cope with the stimulus are fed back into the system and compared with the adaptation level and its gradient to the focal stimulus. If the effort is not sufficient to cope with the stimulus, the coping mechanisms will be further activated to produce greater responses..." (Roy and McLeod, p 59, 1981).

Relationships of the Basic Concepts to Person, Environment, Health, and Nursing

Adaptation is a central and unifying concept within the model. The recipient of nursing care is the person as an adaptive system receiving stimuli from the environment in the dimensions of his/her life related to health and illness. These stimuli may be inside or outside the person's zone of adaptation and she/he uses the regulator and cognator subsystems to maintain adaptation in regard to the four adaptive modes. Nursing promotes adaptation in situations of health and illness through the use of the nursing process (Roy, 1970, 1971, 1973, 1980; Roy and McLeod, 1981; Roy and Roberts, 1981).

INTERNAL ANALYSIS

Underlying Assumptions

Roy (1980) identifies eight basic assumptions of the Adaptation Model of Nursing. These assumptions are:

1. The person is a biopsychosocial being.
2. The person is in constant interaction with a changing environment.
3. To cope with a changing world, the person uses both innate and acquired mechanisms, which are biologic, psychologic, and social in origin.
4. Health and illness are one inevitable dimension of the person's life.
5. To respond positively to environmental changes, the person must adapt.
6. The person's adaptation is a function of the stimulus he is exposed to and his adaptation level.
7. The person's adaptation level is such that it comprises a zone indicating the range of stimulation that will lead to a positive response.
8. The person is conceptualized as having four modes of adaptation: physiologic needs, self-concept, role function, interdependence relations (pp 180-182).

Roy (1976d) also proposes two further assumptions in regard to the self-concept mode. These assumptions are:

1. The self-concept arises out of perception and is the product of social reaction.
2. Self-concept has a predictable effect on behavior.

The soundness of the assumptions can be assessed using the three levels of assumptions identified by Fox (1970). First level assumptions are the soundest and have their foundations in previous research. Second level assumptions are those which stem from general theory, particularly if there are empirical data available to indicate that the theory has substance. Third level assumptions are based on the personal experience of the researcher and others.

Assumptions 1 through 7 of the model can be classified as second level assumptions. These assumptions stem from theory in physiologic psychology, psychology, sociology, and nursing and there are empirical data to indicate that this general theory base has substance. The two additional assumptions can also be classified as second level assumptions and are derived from theories of growth and development, motivation, and learning.

Assumption 8 is the weakest and would be classified as third level; it is based on the experience of Roy and others. Roy (1970, 1980) studied and analyzed 500 samples of patient behaviors collected by nursing students. From the analyses Roy proposed that man has four adaptive modes.

The assumptions can also be analyzed to determine what type of statements they are. Reynolds (1971) describes two basic types of statements—existence statements and relational statements. Existence statements claim the existence of phenomena referred to by a concept while relational statements describe a relationship between concepts. Relational statements may be further classified as associational or causal. "The heart of scientific knowledge is expressed in relational statements" (p 69). Only relations may be tested, not isolated facts (Kerlinger, 1973). Of the eight basic assumptions in the model, assumptions 1 through 5 are existence statements. Assumptions 6 and 7 and the two additional assumptions are associational statements.

Roy identifies many propositions in relation to the regulator and cognator mechanisms and the self-concept, role function, and interdependence modes (Roy and McLeod, 1981; Roy and Roberts, 1980). These propositions have varying degrees of support from general theory and empirical data. The majority of the propositions are relational statements. They can be used to generate testable hypotheses.

Central Components of the Model

The central components of the Roy Adaptation Model of Nursing are the concepts of person, adaptation, nursing, health-illness, and environment. One way to examine these concepts is to classify them according to Dubin's (1978) types of units. It is essential to point out that these units are properties of things rather than the things themselves. Therefore, the classification system is not applicable to all of the concepts, e.g., person, nursing, and environment. It is possible to classify the concept of adaptive system in this manner. The concept of adaptive system would be a summative unit, i.e., it is global and it stands for the entire complex thing. As a summative unit it draws together a number of different properties and gives them a label that highlights one of the more important properties.

This classification of units can be applied to the concepts of adaptation level and adaptation zone. Both concepts would be enumerative units. Enumerative units are universal—they are always present in the thing and they can never have a zero value or a sample member who does not exhibit that characteristic. Both adaptation level and adaptation zone would also be relational units in that they are properties which are derivable from at least two other properties. Adaptation level, which sets up the adaptation zone, is the pooled effect of focal, contextual, and residual stimuli. Thus, adaptation level and adaptation zone derive from the person-environment interaction. Health-illness can also be classified using Dubin's types of units. Health-illness would also be an enumerative unit because it is an inevitable dimension of the person's life.

Relative Importance of the Components

The components of the model which receive the most emphasis by Roy are the concepts of the person as an adaptive system and adaptation. These concepts are discussed by Roy in detail and in depth. The concepts of the person as an adaptive system and adaptation are also the concepts which have received the most attention in the clarification and refinement of the model. Adaptation is viewed in this discussion as the central and unifying concept of the model. It is the concept of adaptation which links the person and nursing.

The nursing process has been clearly delineated within the model although it has received less attention within the model than the concepts of person and adaptation. This is particularly true in Roy's most recent writings. Health-illness and environment receive little attention within the model; this author believes that health-illness in particular needs to receive more attention and clarification.

Analysis of Consistency

In assessing the internal consistency of the model, one needs to determine if the concepts are clearly and consistently defined, if the relationships between the concepts are clear and consistent, and if the assumptions are consistent with the concepts and the relationships between the concepts.

The concepts of person, adaptation, and nursing are clearly defined within the model. However, there appear to be some inconsistencies in the definitions of person and nursing. Roy defines the person as a living, open system, negentropic, and exchanging matter and energy with the environment. However, she also defines the person as a biopsychosocial being, a whole made up of parts, and a system which adapts to a changing environment. This mechanistic, rather closed view of the person seems inconsistent with her description of person as an open system.

In her definition of adaptation nursing, Roy states that nursing views the person as having modes of adapting to a changing environment. This definition is inconsistent with her refinement of the concept of the person as an adaptive system.

In her earlier works Roy (1970, 1976b) described the person as having four modes or ways of adapting or coping, i.e., the physiologic needs, self-concept, role function, and interdependence. These modes were seen by Roy as ways of adapting to a changing environment. In her most recent work Roy describes the person as having mechanisms for coping, i.e., the regulator and cognator mechanisms are the ways or methods of adapting or coping. These mechanisms of coping act in relation to or are effected through the four modes (Roy and McLeod, 1981). The definition of adaptation nursing should thus reflect this change in the concept of the person as an adaptive system.

Health is not specifically defined within the model although the health-illness continuum is defined. This continuum uses both the terms health and wellness. Environment is defined using a dictionary definition. Further work is underway to clarify environment as distinct from internal stimuli (Roy and Roberts, 1981).

The relationships among the concepts vary in clarity but there are no discrepancies or contradictions within the relationships. The relationships among person, adaptation, and nursing are clear. The person adapts and nursing promotes this adaptation in situations of health and illness. For each person the relationship between health-illness is an inevitable dimension of life; it is not clear, however, how this dimension is differentiated from other dimensions of the person's life. Adaptation is seen as leading to a higher level wellness (health) and an adaptive response is seen as promoting the integrity of the individual in regard to the general goals of survival, growth, reproduction, and mastery. The question is then raised: Is higher level wellness or integrity the result of adaptation in all situations or only in those of health and illness?

The basic assumptions of the model are consistent with the definitions of the concepts and the relationships between them. An inconsistency appears with regard to the person as an open system and the more mechanistic, closed view of the person suggested in the assumptions.

Analysis of Adequacy

Hardy (1974) describes two criteria for assessing the adequacy of a model—meaning and logical adequacy, and operational and empirical adequacy. In assessing meaning and logical adequacy one needs to examine the validity of the assumptions and the validity of the meaning attributed to the concepts, i.e., are they defined in a manner similar to that used by other scientists in the area? In addition, one needs to examine the logic of the theoretical system.

Person, adaptation, and nursing are clearly defined and explained in detail within the model. Although each of the concepts has aspects which are unique to the model, each has aspects which are similar to those used by other scientists in the area.

The cognator and regulator as adaptive mechanisms are unique to the model although there is support for the concept of adaptive mechanisms in the conceptions of persons specified by other scientists. The idea of persons having four adaptive modes is also unique to the model.

Two aspects of nursing are unique to the model—the two-level assessment in the nursing process and intervention as manipulation of stimuli. The two-level assessment provides for the assessment of patient behavior/responses and the stimuli to which the patient is responding. This is appropriate to a model which focuses on the person responding to stimuli present due to his/her position on the health-illness continuum. The specifications within the model of nursing intervention as the manipulation of focal, contextual, and residual stimuli raises a question. Can residual stimuli be manipulated without manipulating the person? Roy clearly states that the manipulation of stimuli is different from manipulating people; an example would serve to clarify this point (Roy and Roberts, 1981).

The concept of adaptation as process and product draws upon the definitions of other theorists—Dohrenwend (1961), Lazarus (1966), Mechanic (1970), and Selye (1978) who define adaptation as a process and Helson (1964) who defines adaptation as a product. The model combines the various aspects of these definitions in a logical manner and maintains a high degree of intersubjectivity with the original definitions of these theorists.

The logical adequacy of the model can be assessed by examining the relationships between the concepts. Most of the relationships are clearly described by Roy. There are no apparent discrepancies or contradictions.

In assessing operational and empirical adequacy one asks the following questions: Can the concepts be measured? Do operational definitions reflect theoretical concepts? And, does the evidence support the theory? (Hardy, 1974) As a broad model for nursing, the adaptation model does not operationally define the major concepts. However, general propositions have been developed in the model and from the propositions it is possible to deduce testable hypotheses. Concepts contained in these hypotheses could be operationally defined in a manner which would be theoretically consistent with the concepts and would be measurable. Testable hypotheses have been derived from the model (Hill and Roberts, 1981). As these are tested there will be evidence (empirical data) against which to judge portions of the model.

One can further assess the adequacy of the model by examining its scope and complexity. Ellis (1968) considers scope and complexity to be characteristics of significant theory. The Adaptation Model of Nursing is broad in scope in that it can be applied to all situations of health or illness in any setting. The model is also complex, i.e., it deals with multiple concepts and relationships and the individual concepts are complex. This is particularly true of the concepts of man and adaptation.

Ellis (1968) identifies two further criteria for assessing the adequacy of a model—its usefulness for practice and its capability for generating new information. The Roy Adaptation Model with its clearly defined nursing process would be useful in guiding clinical practice. This usefulness for clinical practice will be discussed in more depth later. It would also appear that the model is capable of generating new information. As hypotheses based on the model are developed and tested, new information will be generated.

EXTERNAL THEORY ANALYSIS

Relationship to Nursing Research

The usefulness of a model for research depends on the ability of the model to generate testable hypotheses. Dickoff and James (1968a) state that a viable theory cannot exist without research. To test theory it is necessary to develop hypotheses which can be tested. These hypotheses must state relationships (Kerlinger, 1973). Within her model Roy has generated a number of general propositions (Roy and McLeod, 1981; Roy and Roberts, 1981). From these general propositions specific propositions or hypotheses can be developed and tested. Roy cites examples of such testable hypotheses which she states are relevant for specifying prescriptions for practice. Hill and Roberts (1981) have also demonstrated the development of testable hypotheses from the model. The testing of such hypotheses would also generate data which can be used to validate or support the model. To date there has been little research in this area.

The concepts identified by Roy (1970) provide a model for the long term process of observation and classification of facts which would lead to postulates regarding: the occurrence of adaptation problems, coping mechanisms, and interventions based on laws derived from factors making up the response potential, i.e., focal, contextual, and residual stimuli. There is a beginning outline of a typology of adaptation problems or nursing diagnosis and work is continuing in this area (Roy, 1973, 1975a, 1975b, 1976a). There is a need to develop an organization of categories of interventions which fit within the model (Roy and Roberts, 1981). Research and testing is needed in both these areas. Some work has been done regarding the coping mechanisms. General propositions have been developed which need to be tested (Roy and McLeod, 1981).

Research has been done using the Adaptation Model of Nursing. A group of graduate students tested the model in a number of practice situations. A nursing process tool was developed as an adaptation of the design presented by Roy (1971). This tool was used to test the model in episodic settings, such as a variety of units in different hospitals, and in distributive settings, such as physicians' offices, outpatient clinics and industrial health settings. Although there were some problems in the use of the tool, the students concluded that the model provided a good framework for ordering a variety of observations and was flexible enough to be used in both episodic and distributive settings (Wagner, 1976). This study provides empirical support for the model with regard to the process of assessment within the four adaptive modes. Roy (1980) stated that a pilot research study in 1971 and a survey research study in 1976-1977 led to some tentative confirmations of the model. However, Roy has not further described these studies.

Some research has been conducted on the model to date, and thus it seems that the model can be useful in research. The model does generate many testable hypotheses related to practice and theory.

Relationship to Nursing Education

The Adaptation Model has demonstrated its usefulness in education. The model is currently in use at Mount St. Mary's College, Department of Nursing (Roy, 1973, 1979) and it has been used in a geriatric nurse practitioner program (Brower and Baker, 1976). The curriculum at Mount St. Mary's clearly demonstrates the relationship of nursing theory to nursing education. There are three vertical strands which run throughout the curriculum. These include two theory strands—the adapting person and health-illness—and one practice strand—nursing management. There are two horizontal strands built into the curriculum— nursing process and student adaptation/leadership. The horizontal strands help the theory and practice of the vertical strands. All strands within the curriculum build in complexity from one level to the next (Roy, 1979). Also, the model allows for increasing knowledge in both the areas of theory and practice (Roy, 1973).

According to Roy (1973, 1979), the model leads students to a clear view of the distinct purpose of nursing, i.e., promoting adaptation to lead to a higher-level wellness. The model also distinguishes nursing science and medical science and the content of these areas is taught in separate courses. Roy (1979) believes that the curriculum based on this model helps students with theory development. Students are taught to test out theory and to develop new theoretical insights. Brower and Baker (1976) state that the adaptation model integrates nursing theory, thereby decreasing students' anxiety. They also state that the model provides for some overlap as well as distinction between medicine and nursing.

Relationship to Professional Nursing Practice

Brower and Baker (1976) consider the Adaptation Model useful for nursing practitioners because it outlines the features of the discipline and provides direction for practice as well as for education and research. The model considers goals, values, the client, and practitioner interventions, i.e., it is situation-producing.

The model can indeed be classified as situation-producing theory. It is theory which is designed to allow for the production of desired situations and as such has three essential ingredients: 1) goal content specified as the aim for activity; 2) prescriptions for activity to realize the goal content; and, 3) a survey list (Dickoff and James, 1968b; Dickoff, James and Wiedenbach, 1968). The goal of the model is the person's adaptation in the four adaptive modes in situations of health and illness and the prescriptions or interventions are the manipulation of stimuli. These prescriptions can be obtained by listing practice-related hypotheses generated by the model (Roy, 1970, 1973, 1976b, 1980; Roy and Roberts, 1981).

The survey list contains six items: agency, patiency, framework, terminus, procedure, and dynamics (Dickoff and James, 1968b; Dickoff, James and Wiedenbach, 1968). Roy (1974) deals with each of these items. Patiency and agency are both the patient as an adaptive system, the framework can be any setting, any time with man in situations of health and illness, the terminus is the goal of the model, the procedure is the nursing process, and the dynamics or energy source is the patient's adaptive mechanisms.

The nursing process is well developed for use in a practice setting. The two-level assessment leads to the identification of adaptation problems or nursing diagnoses. There is a beginning typology of nursing diagnosis and there is continuing work in this area (Roy, 1973, 1975a, 1975b, 1976a; Roy and Roberts, 1981). Intervention is based specifically on the model but work is needed to organize categories of nursing interventions.

The model has been used in practice by a number of nurses. Students who used the model as a research project found some overlap in aspects of self-concept, role function, and interdependence. They also found the nursing process lengthy and repetitious; it took much time to complete. There are no major deterrents to its use in inpatient settings except in intensive care units where there were rapid changes in the patient's condition. They did find it easier to work with the model in outpatient settings such as clinics and physicians' offices (Wagner, 1976).

Galligan (1979) used the model to care for young, hospitalized children. She found that the Adaptation Model provided a means for guiding nurses in a more conscious effort to assist the child during hospitalization. The model provided a system which considered physical needs as only one aspect of care and provided an organization for focusing on psychosocial needs. It also provided for reevaluation of the child's case during his/her hospital stay.

The model has also been used in a community setting where the client received care in the home. It was possible using the model to assess needs, prioritize, set goals, and intervene efficiently and effectively (Schmitz, 1980).

SUMMARY

It has been shown that the Roy Adaptation Model is a complex model that deals with multiple concepts and relationships. The individual concepts are also complex. Within this complexity there are a few inconsistencies in the definition of the concepts and some vagueness in the description of the relationships between concepts. The model, however, is broad in scope and can be applied in many situations. In practice the model has been found very useful in inpatient settings, outpatient settings and in the community. The model has also been found useful in education. Although the model has not been used widely in research, it is capable of generating new information. The propositions can be used to deduce testable hypotheses. Roy's model makes a significant contribution to nursing's body of knowledge.

REFERENCES

Brower HTF, Baker BJ: The Roy adaptation model: Using the adaptation model in a practitioner curriculum. Nursing Outlook, Vol 24, No 18, pp 686-689, 1976

Dickoff J, James P: Researching research's role in theory development. Nursing Research, Vol 17, No 3, pp 204-206, 1968a

Dickoff J, James P: A theory of theories: A position paper. Nursing Research, Vol 17, No 3, pp 197-203, 1968b

Dickoff J, James P, Wiedenbach E: Theory in a practice discipline, part I, practice oriented theory. Nursing Research, Vol 17, No 5, pp 413-435, 1968

Dohrenwend BP: The social psychological nature of stress: A framework for causal inquiry. Journal of Abnormal and Social Psychology, Vol 62, No 2, pp 294-302, 1961

Dubin R: Theory Building. The Free Press, New York, 1978

Duffey M, Muhlenkamp AF: A framework for theory analysis. Nursing Outlook, Vol 22, No 9, pp 570-574, 1974

Ellis R: Characteristics of significant theories. Nursing Research, Vol 17, No 3, pp 217-222, 1968

Fox D: Fundamentals of Research in Nursing, 2nd ed. Appleton-Century-Crofts, New York, 1970

Galligan AC: Using Roy's concept of adaptation to care for young children. The American Journal of Maternal Child Nursing, Vol 4, No 1, pp 24-28, 1979

Hardy ME: Theories: Components, development, evaluation. Nursing Research, Vol 23, No 2, pp 100-107, 1974

Helson H: Adaptation-Level Theory: An Experimental and Systematic Approach to Behavior. Harper & Row Publishers, Inc., New York, 1964

Hill BJ, Roberts CS: Formal theory construction: An example of the process. In Roy C, Roberts SL (eds): Theory Construction in Nursing: An Adaptation Model, Prentice-Hall, Inc., Englewood Cliffs, New Jersey, 1981

Kerlinger FN: Foundations of Behavioral Research, 2nd ed. Holt, Rinehart & Winston, New York, 1973

Lazarus RS: Psychological Stress and the Coping Process. McGraw-Hill Book Co., New York, 1966

Mechanic D: Some problems in developing a social psychology of adaptation to stress. In McGrath J (ed): Social and Psychological Factors in Stress, Holt, Rinehart & Winston, New York, 1970

Reynolds PD: A Primer in Theory Construction. The Bobbs-Merrill Co., Inc., Indianapolis, Indiana, 1971

Roy C: Adaptation: A conceptual framework for nursing. Nursing Outlook, Vol 18, No 3, pp 42-45, 1970

Roy C: Adaptation: A basis for nursing practice. Nursing Outlook, Vol 19, No 4, pp 254-257, 1971

Roy C: Adaptation: Implications for curriculum change. Nursing Outlook, Vol 21, No 3, pp 163-168, 1973

Roy C: The Roy adaptation model. In Riehl JP, Roy C (eds): Conceptual Models for Nursing Practice, Appleton-Century-Crofts, New York, 1974

Roy C: A diagnostic classification system for nursing. Nursing Outlook, Vol 23, No 2, pp 90-94, 1975a

Roy C: The impact of nursing diagnosis. AORN, Vol 21, No 6, pp 1023-1030, 1975b

Roy C: The impact of nursing diagnosis. Nursing Digest, pp 67-69, Summer, 1976a

Roy C: Introduction to Nursing: An Adaptation Model. Prentice-Hall, Inc., Englewood Cliffs, New Jersey, 1976b

Roy C: The Roy adaptation model: Comment. Nursing Outlook, Vol 24, No 11, pp 690-691, 1976c

Roy C: The Roy adaptation model: Past, present, and future. Taped at Wayne State University, Detroit, Michigan, 1976d

Roy C: Relating nursing theory to education: A new era. Nurse Educator, Vol IV, No 2, pp 16-21, 1979

Roy C: The Roy adaptation model. In Riehl JP, Roy C (eds): Conceptual Models for Nursing Practice, 2nd ed, Appleton-Century-Crofts, New York, 1980

Roy C, Roberts SL (eds): Theory Construction in Nursing: An Adaptation Model. Prentice-Hall, Inc., Englewood Cliffs, New Jersey, 1981

Roy C, McLeod D: Theory of the person as an adaptive system. In Roy C, Roberts SL (eds): Theory Construction in Nursing: An Adaptation Model, Prentice-Hall, Inc., Englewood Cliffs, New Jersey, 1981

Schmitz M: The Roy adaptation model: Application in a community setting. In Riehl JP, Roy C (eds): Conceptual models for Nursing Practice, 2nd ed, Appleton-Century-Crofts, New York, 1980

Selye H: The Stress of Life. McGraw-Hill Book Co., New York, 1978

Wagner P: The Roy adaptation model: Testing the adaptation model in practice. Nursing Outlook, Vol 24, No 11, pp 662-685, 1976

11

PATERSON AND ZDERAD:
A HUMANISTIC NURSING MODEL

Shirley Cloutier Laffrey & Suzanne H. Brouse

INTRODUCTION

After a number of years of clinical practice and teaching, Josephine Paterson and Loretta Zderad became increasingly dissatisfied with the ability of positivistic science to address phenomena they considered relevant to nursing in its current stage of development. Motivated by their individual questions in nursing situations and their beliefs about the nature of person, and strongly influenced by the literary works of Husserl, Marcel, and Buber, their world view has evolved since 1960. They continue to examine, question, explore, and analyze their own and other nurses' experiences in an attempt to identify those phenomena of importance to nursing.

Humanistic nursing has evolved out of this questioning and exploring process, and is described by Paterson and Zderad (p 18, 1976) as a "kind of nursing practice and its theoretical foundations." The term Humanistic Nursing was chosen to signify nursing's human foundations and meaning and to direct nursing's development by exploring and expanding its relation to its human context.

The initial intent was not to develop a theory, but rather to develop a method or process to creatively conceptualize their nursing experiences. Their initial commitment to creatively conceptualize nursing constructs developed into Nursology, a phenomenological approach to studying nursing itself. Through analysis and synthesis of the nursing constructs considered important in nursing practice, the theorists hope to "point the direction for nursing's development" (Paterson and Zderad, p 15, 1976) and in this way lead to a science of nursing.

View Of Theory

Paterson and Zderad espouse a view of theory different from that of many other current nurse-theorists. Their conceptualization of theory as the articulated vision of experience is derived from Laing (1967). Vision refers to a philosophical perspective or a particular world view. Experience refers to the nurse's existential encounter with the patient and with others in the health-illness community. Articulated means that the conceptualized experience is clearly expressed and connected to form a systematic whole.

Use Of Phenomenology

The phenomenological method is used by Paterson and Zderad to describe the nature of nursing as experienced by individual nurses. Phenomenology is the descriptive study of phenomena (Paterson and Zderad, 1976) and is seen as a way of dealing with the foundational questions of all human endeavors (Stewart, 1974). Natanson (p 25, 1973) notes that the phenomenological method is a "way of posing questions and searching for answers." This requires a recognition that phenomena are immediately given states of affairs rather than empirical posits, and attention must be given to the phenomena in both descriptive and analytical terms (Natanson, p 25). Natanson emphasizes that, although phenomenologists differ greatly in their approach and purposes, an essential commonality can be recognized. "For the phenomenologist, the experienced world is thematized as 'experience-of,' the necessary conditions for 'experience-of' are inspected and elucidated, and the activity of consciousness in relation to its thermatizable possibilities is explored" (Natanson, p 26). This illustrates the intimate relationship between the method and the experience being studied. Its development by Husserl, the father of phenomenology, was aimed at facilitating "an original intuition of things themselves and a return to immediate and original data of consciousness" (Zeitlin, p 144, 1973). This requires looking at the world differently. All previous judgments and positions must be put aside (bracketed) and experiences are seen through a neutral attitude. One experiences "the thing itself," putting aside all previous notions of the experience.

In humanistic nursing practice theory, the thing itself is the existentially experienced nursing situation (Paterson and Zderad, p 6, 1976). The theorists in dialogue together and with groups of nurses reflected on, explored, and questioned nursing situational experiences. They recognized the need to know how man experienced his existence. The study of the nursing event itself and its conceptualization is an application of phenomenology.

The phenomenological method is complementary to and operates at qualitatively different levels than empirical science. Phenomenology deals with questions which empirical science cannot answer; questions which are "either presupposed by empirical science or unavailable to its procedures." "Empiricism begins where phenomenology leaves off" (Natanson, p 33, 1973).

In Paterson and Zderad's nursology, the observer perceives an experience or event intuitively and spontaneously, and knows the phenomenon as it is experienced. Pre-conceived labels or judgments about the event are held in abeyance. Then, as many instances of the experiencing as possible are described. After a large number of descriptions are gathered from as many nurses as possible, these data are analyzed, compared, synthesized, and further conceptualized. The latter requires a shift in focus from the parts to the whole. Since individual nurse theorists may differ in their conceptualization of the whole, Paterson and Zderad envision the potential for development of many levels of theory (Zderad, 1978).

BASIC CONSIDERATIONS

Person

Buber's existential view of person serves as the base for humanistic nursing's concept of person. Person is viewed as an "incarnate being always becoming in relation with men and things in a world of time and space" (Paterson and Zderad, p 19, 1976). It is through the body that a person interacts with the world of person and things, affects the world, and is affected by it. Through the body each person develops a unique personal private world, the here and now. Person is distinguished from other beings by a capacity for knowing self and the inner world, and by a capability for self-reflection and becoming more.

Special characteristics of relating derived from Buber (1958) are described by Paterson and Zderad, and form the basis for humanistic nursing theory. The first, *I-Thou* relating, is the intuitive, intersubjective dialogue that occurs when person merges with otherness. Each recognizes self apart from the other, is aware of the other's uniqueness, and offers the other authentic presence, allowing authentic presence of the other with the self. Authenticity involves auditory, olfactory, oral, visual, and kinesthetic responses, each conveying unique meaning to person's consciousness. Awareness of these sensations and responses informs the person of the quality of presence with the other. Each becomes more through I-Thou relating (Paterson and Zderad, 1976).

The second characteristic of relating described by the theorists is "I-It" relating. I-It relating is subject-object relating. As I-Thou relating is experienced by each individual, each reflects on the process, interprets and gives meaning to the experience. I-It relating is similar to the way persons interact with objects, but with an essential difference. An object is open to scrutiny while a person, as object, can either make self knowable to the other or set up barriers to objectification. A person may remain silent or deliberately conceal ideas, feelings, or qualities.

A third characteristic of relating described by Paterson and Zderad is "We" relating. This permits the phenomenon of community and of adult contributions to the world. Community is defined as "two or more persons struggling toward a center" (Paterson and Zderad, p 131, 1976).

Uniqueness is a universal characteristic of the human species. Therefore, only the person can describe and choose his/her own angular, biased, or shaded reality. Human beings are also characterized by a commonality with others, a uniqueness and commonality constantly interplaying and affecting each other. Although influenced by habit and unconscious motivation, as well as potentials and limitations, persons are and become more through their choices. The here-and-now person became because of choosing certain alternatives and actualizing certain opportunities. Because of human nondeterminedness, alternatives chosen may be experienced as contradictory and inconsistent. Human nature is perceived by Paterson and Zderad as contradictory and conflictual. On one side is ideal spirituality and on the other, materialistic animalism. Recognition of this dualism in humanness permits acceptance of one's own and others' vices and virtues.

This conceptualization of person as applying to both nurse and patient is emphasized, although more attention is given to the nurse. Relating between the nurse and patient has special characteristics not necessarily present in other transactions. Recognition is given to the patient's vulnerability. The openness of the nurse is an openness to a "person-with-needs" and his/her availability is an availability-in-a-helping-way. A type of professional reserve contributes to a different quality of intimacy, flowing through a filter of professional tact (Paterson and Zderad, p 31, 1976).

Nursing

Nursing is conceptualized as a lived human act, a response to a human situation. This response is purposely directed toward nurturing the well-being and more-being of a person with perceived needs related to the health/illness quality of living (Paterson and Zderad, p 19, 1976). Thus a boundary is drawn around nursing in the sense that it is restricted to the health/illness situation. Additionally, nursing is seen as a response to a call for help. Paterson and Zderad go on to say that nursing is a meeting of persons, patient and nurse, with a goal or expectation in mind. "The patient expects to receive help and the nurse expects to give help" (Paterson and Zderad, p 27, 1976).

Nursing is studied phenomenologically by studying the thing itself. Paterson (p 51, 1978) describes the nursing thing itself as "the act of nursing, the intersubjective transactional relation, the dialogue experience, lived in concert between persons where comfort and nurturance prod mutual unfolding." Paterson's use of *transaction* follows from that of Dewey (1949) and focuses on the individual's aware knowing of his/her part in a two-way interaction (Zderad, 1982). The use of *intersubjective* refers to the shared between of two or more human beings (Paterson and Zderad, 1976). The goal of nursing, therefore, is well-being and more-being and mutual unfolding for both nurse and patient.

The dialogical quality of nursing is emphasized; nursing is viewed as a transaction between persons (Paterson, 1978). The dialogue between nurse and patient is also described as "flowing like a stream" (Paterson and Zderad, p 23, 1976). The between is the basic relation through which nursing can occur (Paterson and Zderad, p 24, 1976).

Humanistic Nursing

A central concept in the work of Paterson and Zderad is humanistic nursing, a special kind of nursing. This is defined as a "responsible searching transactional relationship whose meaningfulness demands conceptualization founded on a nurse's existential awareness of self and of the other" (Paterson and Zderad, p 3, 1976). Humanistic nursing goes beyond nursing which "aims at the development of human potential, at well-being and more-being" (p 14) to "point the future directions for nursing's development" (p 15).

Health

Although the term *health* is used repeatedly by the theorists, no actual definiton of health is provided. One can infer from their description of well-being and more-being that health is conceptualized as somewhat more than the freedom from disease. The theorists acknowledge that health is commonly accepted as the aim of nursing. They follow this with the statement that nursing's concern is said to be "not merely with a person's well-being but with his more-being; with helping him become more as humanly possible in his particular life situation" (Paterson and Zderad, p 12, 1976).

Health is further used in the context of the "health/illness" quality of life and the "health/nursing" situation. The use of these terms may be an attempt to define the special context in which nursing occurs and the nurse's special role of helper to another human being who needs help.

Environment

Paterson and Zderad view person as actually living in two worlds, an angular, inner world, also described as a biased or shaded reality, and the objective world of persons and things. Openness to and acceptance of the other's inner world is essential for true interaction between persons. Family, friends, and significant others are an important part of each person's world. Nurse-patient transactions occur within an intra-and interdisciplinary milieu in the complex health care system. Transactions are subject to influence of the constantly changing personnel, roles, and functions (Paterson and Zderad, p 38, 1976). While two persons may share a situation, objects enhance or inhibit person-to-person interactions because of the different meanings ascribed to them by each person.

Time is experienced in the real world not only as measured time, but also as time lived by patient and nurse in their private worlds. When dialogue between persons is truly intersubjective it is characterized by synchrony, or shared clock time and private lived time. The nurse and patient experience a harmony with the rhythm of the dialogue or timing of the flow, and pace their call and response to each other (Paterson and Zderad, 1976).

Measured space (the physical setting) and space as experienced by two persons affect human dialogue. Really being with another involves knowing the other in that person's lived space. Lived space and lived time are seen as interrelated. A person feels more comfortable in a particular space over time and often begins to assume a sense of ownership, "The person feels he belongs in the place and the place belongs to him" (Paterson and Zderad, p 38, 1976).

Interrelations Among the Concepts, Person, Health, Environment, and Nursing

In order to discuss the interrelationship of person, environment, health, and nursing, the rather unique definition of nursing, the implied definition of environment, and the lack of a clear definition of health in humanistic nursing theory must be acknowledged. Nursing is defined as an intersubjective transaction between nurse as helper and a patient with special needs. The goal of nursing is nurturance of well-being and more-being. The derived definition of environment includes interactions between the private inner world of the individuals, and the world of other persons and things, in both clock and lived time and space. Health is not clearly defined, nor does it occupy a central position as in other nursing theories. The nursing act is always related, however, to the health-illness quality of human condition, to a person's living and dying.

Nursing Process

The assessment phase of the nursing process is seen as the nurse "constantly assesses the patient's capabilities and needs..." (Paterson and Zderad, p 17, 1976). The intervention phase is most clearly seen in the theorists' statement that "the nurse coexperiences and supports the process from his (the patient's) point of view, thus nurturing his human potential for responsible choosing" (Paterson and Zderad, p 17, 1976). Both of these can logically be seen as nursing interventions. Intersubjective relating (being with) is emphasized to a much greater extent in humanistic nursing theory than physical care (doing with). Being with is described as intuitive experiencing, yet the meeting of nurse and patient is said to be goal-directed within the context of the patient's health/illness needs. Both nurse and patient have expectations; the patient expects to be helped and the nurse expects to give help. In this sense, the planning phase of the nursing process can be assumed at least for the goal-directed aspects of the nurse-patient interaction. The theorists emphasize the necessity for bracketing one's world view, values, perspectives, and judgments so as not to impose these on the nurse-patient intersubjective relating. It is not made clear how this bracketing or holding aside of one's judgment and perspective allows for the interaction to be goal-directed.

The evaluation phase of the nursing process is not addressed directly but can be inferred from the I-It characteristic of relating in which the nurse and patient each reflect on and validate the I-Thou relating. This leads the way to "working through the possible meanings of the experience and to speculating about outcomes or alternative future nursing actions and behaviors" (Paterson and Zderad, p 17, 1976).

Although in addressing *being with* and *doing with,* one can infer a wide variety of nursing activities within the humanistic nursing framework, the major emphasis is placed on intersubjective relating between nurse and patient.

A clearer description of how the major concepts in the model relate to the provision of physical care would provide a valuable addition to humanistic nursing.

CENTRAL COMPONENTS OF THE MODEL

The basic concepts included in Humanistic Nursing Theory are: nurse, patient (nursed), interhuman relating, well-being, and more-being.

The major question of concern to Paterson and Zderad in developing their theory of nursing was the what, why, and how of nursing. Humanistic nursing is described by them variously as an approach to the conceptualization of nursing acts as these are experienced by nurses, a nursing practice theory, and a metatheory, defined as "ontological inquiry from which theory may be derived" (Paterson and Zderad, p 132, 1976).

Nurse

The nurse's self-awareness, in-touchness, self-acceptance, and actualization allows him/her to share with others so they can become in relation to the nurse. The nursing act is a behavioral expression of the nurse's state of being (Paterson and Zderad, p 13, 1976). The nursing goal is an expression of authentic commitment directed toward nurturing human potential. The nurse is open to the patient, not as a thing, but as a presence, a human being with potentials. She/he sees in the human being a form or possibility for well-being and more-being (Paterson and Zderad, p 101, 1976).

Patient (Nursed)

The patient is defined as incarnate person with all of the characteristics of person being and becoming. Patient is a specific definition of person as one with needs related to the health-illness quality of life.

Interhuman Relating

The nurse enters into genuine relation with the patient. The caring, nursing skills, and hope bring forth the form; the patient's potential for well-being and more-being is realized. The patient (nursed) participates as an active subject to actualize the potential within, and also sees a form or possibility in the nurse for nursing (help and support). The patient responds to the nurse to bring forth that possibility (Paterson and Zderad, 1976). The interhuman relating is described as a particular kind of flowing, a between. Each knows the other and more of himself in this relating. The relating is a combination of I-Thou relating and I-It relating.

Both are essential components of interhuman relating. The nurse relates as an authentic presence, allowing authentic presence of the patient. Neither superimposes or decides about the other. Each becomes more through the relationship. The nurse steps back and reflects on the I-Thou relationship, allowing interpretation of the experience. The nurse analyzes, considers relationships between components, synthesizes themes and patterns, and then conceptualizes... "a sequential view of this past lived reality" (Paterson and Zderad, p 79, 1976).

The interhuman relating process is a complex phenomenon which can be described only in sequence, but which in reality occurs all-at-once as each participant experiences I-Thou and I-It relating simultaneously. The call and response (patient's call for help and nurse's response or giving of help) occur sequentially and also simultaneously. The patient's request is a call for help and, at the same time, a response to the nurse's availability or offer to be of help. The nurse's response is a call to him/her for a particular kind of response. All-at-once is proposed by Paterson and Zderad to reflect the complexities that exist in the nursing situation.

Well-Being/More-Being

Well-being and more-being are viewed by Paterson and Zderad as the aim of nursing and as the potential or form seen within the patient. Through the experience and relationships with others the person becomes ever more the person she/he has the human capacity to be. Nursing's concern is with more-being, with helping the person become more as humanly possible in his/her particular life situation.

The basic question addressed by the theorists is the what, why, and how of nursing. Well-being and more-being offer a perspective for viewing the "why" of nursing; intersubjective relating is concerned with the "how" of nursing; and all-at-once provides a way of conceptualizing the "what" of nursing.

The relationships among these concepts are shown in Figure 11.1.

Nursing is an interhuman process directed toward well-being and more-being. Both nurse and patient are viewed as incarnate man related in a shared situation. Both move toward more-being through interhuman relating.

The theory or model is described as an open framework to allow for many lived nursing worlds to be "explored freely, imaginatively, and creatively in any direction suggested by the dimensions of the framework" (Paterson and Zderad, p 19, 1976). This description of an open framework is very consistent with the theorists' use of the term *metatheory* to describe their "theory." Metatheory is defined by Paterson and Zderad (p 132, 1976) as "transcending theory; ontological inquiry from which theory may be derived."

Underlying Assumptions

A number of assumptions and values can be seen in Paterson and Zderad's approach. The first is that the person is unique.

Health/Illness Situation

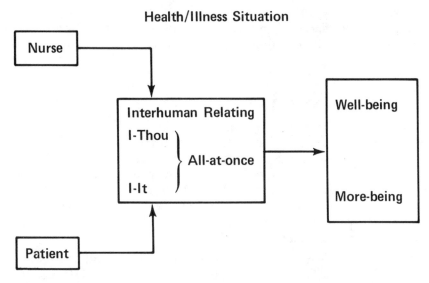

Figure 11.1. Relationships Among Central Concepts in the Model.

From this assumption, the theorists go on to develop their description of the person's uniqueness as a characteristic of the commonality with all other persons.

Secondly, Paterson and Zderad assume "an innate force in human beingness that moves man to come to know his/her own and others' angular views of the world" (Paterson and Zderad, p 15, 1976). A third assumption is that the person has the capacity to move toward ever-increasing human potential. Further, the theorists assume that genuine presence is a positive goal to be strived for, and that the person becomes more through genuine presence. The theorists place a positive value on nursing as an opportunity for development of the human person and lastly, they assume that through describing nursing situations, nurses will better understand and relate to persons as persons. The theory derives clearly and logically from these assumptions and values.

The phenomenological method does not include the use of assumed elements and constructions (Farber, 1966; Paterson and Zderad, 1976). The assumptions and values inherent in Paterson and Zderad's approach to theorizing are in violation with the basic premise of phenomenology. Stewart and Mickunas acknowledge this problem (p 7, 1974), noting that "even a view that a philosophy without presuppositions is possible is itself a pre-supposition." Farber (1966) cautions that the phenomenologist is a cultural product and can never escape totally his/her world view.

INTERNAL ANALYSIS

Analysis of a model must necessarily relate to the purpose for which the model was developed and which it aims to fulfill. Paterson and Zderad developed humanistic nursing theory as an approach or perspective to help nurses become aware of their own practice by describing the nursing acts as they experience them. Out of these descriptions would eventually develop a theory (Paterson and Zderad, 1981).

Descriptive level thory is analogous with Dickoff and James' (1975) factor isolating theory and characterizes a discipline in its early stages of development. Factor isolating theory names factors or concepts, a necessary precondition to developing and testing hypotheses. Phenomenology is therefore viewed as preceding and complementary to positivistic science. This view is supported by Farber (1966) who notes that although one begins with an individual and his/her experience, the phenomenological method must be used in cooperation with other kinds of methods.

Zeitlin (1973) notes a danger in that the phenomenological method provides no independent means of assessing the validity of the individual's judgments about his/her existential conditions and interpretation of the experience. Zeitlin cautions that although the aim is to grasp the meaning of the interaction as seen by the persons involved, this could result in "description in its most superficial sense" (p 182, 1973). Although to attempt more than description in humanistic nursing theory would be premature (Paterson and Zderad, 1981), Paterson and Zderad clearly state the importance of the second level of theory development: that of interrelating the concepts.

Once a theory has been presented to the nursing community it must be subjected to examination and analysis alongside other nursing theories. Given the definition of humanistic nursing theory as articulated vision of experience, and as a metatheory, the usual criteria for evaluation of a theory must be used with caution. The most important question to be answered is: Is the theory significant for nursing?

Terminology

Ellis (1968) suggests that the terminology in which a theory for nursing is couched must be meaningful. A significant theory would use terminology that can be used meaningfully with phenomena observed in nursing. The phenomena studied in humanistic nursing theory are nursing acts themselves, therefore, they are highly significant. The terminology draws heavily on the existential phenomenology literature. This can be confusing and may inhibit the usefulness of the theory for nurses not familiar with that terminology.

Reynolds (1971) discusses shared agreement of concepts in a theory; that is, are the concepts given a meaning similar to the meaning used by other scientists? Paterson and Zderad state that the aim for nursing is the nurturance of well-being and more-being. More-being is defined as being all that one is capable of in one's life situation. This definition is very close to the definition of *health* used by other nurse theorists (Newman, 1979; Parse, 1981; Rogers, 1970). This change in terminology might serve to confuse readers about the meaning of concepts in humanistic nursing theory.

Complexity

Ellis (1968) states that significant theories have complexity. Simple postulations are not particularly valuable if they express only ideas which are readily apparent. Paterson and Zderad have isolated phenomena which occur in person: person interaction; namely, I-Thou and I-It relating all-at-once. They have postulated that well-being and more-being are attained by this relating method. Each of the concepts is very complex and difficult to define precisely or parsimoniously. As the theory continues to develop and as definitions become more parsimonious, there is potential for great complexity in the relationships as well as in the concepts themselves.

Scope

A theory has scope if it "covers and relates a number of smaller generalizations or concepts and provides at least a potential framework for ordering observations about a variety of phenomena" (Ellis, p 181, 1968). "Theory which directs nursing practice must have the scope to cover the whole person" (Ellis, p 182, 1968).

Humanistic nursing theory derives from nursing practice from being with and doing with the patient (Paterson and Zderad, 1976). The theory is said to be concerned with what is basically nursing ... wherever it occurs regardless of its specialized clinical, functional, or sociocultural form" (Paterson and Zderad, p 19, 1976). "Its 'stuff' includes all possible human and interhuman responses" (Paterson and Zderad, p 19, 1976).

The scope seems broad, given the above definition. There is a framework for ordering observations about many nursing phenomena. The "being with" aspect of nursing receives much more attention by these theorists than the "doing with" aspect. The theorists' clinical focus is psychiatric mental health nursing, with much of their clinical theorizing done in this setting. Although they state that physical care (doing with) is a major part of nursing, the main focus of the theory is said to "go beyond physical care" (Paterson and Zderad, p 20, 1976), and to "focus on the person's unique being and becoming in his situation" (Paterson and Zderad, p 20, 1976). In this sense the theory has broad scope, and is relevant for the whole person and for all of nursing. It would be important that a future stage of development address itself to testing relationships empirically in a variety of nursing settings to determine any modifying effects particular settings might have on interhuman relating.

Logical Adequacy

Logical adequacy may be evaluated by examining a theory for discontinuities, discrepancies, and contradictions (Hardy, 1974). Paterson and Zderad have derived their assumptions from the existentialist phenomenological literature, and through this perspective they view the nursing act. The theory follows logically from, and is consistent with, their assumption.

The essential components of the model and their relationships are described. Nurse and patient meet in an intersubjective transaction and move toward well-being and more-being within the health-illness situation in a world of persons and things in time and space. Persons and things may inhibit or enhance the transaction, as well as the ability of each to experience the lived-time and lived-space of the other.

Paterson and Zderad state that both nurse and patient are active participants in humanistic nursing. They also say that humanistic nursing can occur if the patient is unable to be actively involved, but not if the nurse is unwilling or unable to be so (Paterson and Zderad, 1981). This inconsistency presents a possible contradiction in the theory.

Paterson and Zderad see a focus of attention to body parts or specific patient behavior as interfering with the nurse-patient transaction. Their focus is on the "between" as the basic relation through which nursing occurs. Yet, some aspects of the patient's physical status cannot be known or comprehended by the nurse except by deliberate attention or the use of technology. The patient cannot always provide the information verbally but may give behavioral cues. Although Paterson and Zderad acknowledge attention to body parts to be necessary, their emphasis on the "between" implies that attention to the physical aspects of patient care is a barrier to the practice of humanistic nursing.

Testability

The question of testability has been directed to phenomenology in general. "Can reliable, intersubjective, warranted knowledge be attained through the method of . . . a deeply introspective philosophy?" Further, is the method "more than another version of private, idiosyncratic and insulated theorizing" (Natanson, p 32, 1973)? In answer to these questions, Natanson notes that phenomenology cannot present its method or its results in empirically verifiable terms because it does not accept empiricism as an adequate philosophy of the experiential world. Further, the phenomena studied by phenomenologists are either presupposed or not available to empirical methods. Empiricism begins where phenomenology leaves off and presupposes the phenomenological domain (Natanson, p 33, 1973).

Testability is not requisite for use or significance of a theory according to Ellis (1968), but it is desirable. Humanistic nursing theory, while having potential for testability, contains highly abstract concepts which would need to be defined much more precisely if they were to be operationalized. Hypothesis testing was not intended by Paterson and Zderad. Their method has as its goal the description and discovery of meaning to the participants. Confirmation or disconfirmation would require a different methodology.

Contribution to Understanding

Humanistic nursing theory, although not dealing with new phenomena, suggests a new way in which to view and analyze the nursing act. This increases insight and understanding, thus contributing to present nursing knowledge. The framework of the theory suggests new avenues for exploration by nurses and, therefore, Hardy's criteria for evaluation of contribution to understanding (1974).

Usefulness

Ellis (1968) states that usefulness for clinical practice is an essential ingredient for significance of a theory. The strength of humanistic nursing theory lies primarily in its potential for guiding nursing practice. The theory derives out of clinical nursing situations through the process of clinical theorizing (Zderad, 1978). The process of describing what happens in the nursing act is very close to the act itself, therefore highly significant to nursing practice. The theory, defined as articulated vision of experience, is close to the experience out of which it arose. This makes it very useful for nursing practice.

Well-being and more-being are accepted by Paterson and Zderad as fundamental to nursing. The postulation that well-being and more-being are furthered by I-Thou and I-It relating occurring all-at-once is useful for nurses whose aim is to promote the well-being and more-being of their patients. These are global concepts, not measurable, at least with current methods. Additional description of clinical situations in a variety of settings would assist in clarifying the concepts.

Humanistic nursing theory suggests, not only that well-being and more-being will be achieved by I-Thou and I-It relating, but that these are desired and should be pursued. This type of relating, however, may not be possible or even desirable for all patients and nurses all of the time. The theorists concede that this degree of genuine, authentic withness cannot be achieved all of the time, but should be a goal worth striving for (Paterson and Zderad, 1976). Analysis of the forces in the patient, nurse, and environment that modify the nurse-patient relating process would be helpful in understanding this more clearly.

EXTERNAL ANALYSIS

Relationship to Research

The phenomenological method is proposed as a descriptive approach for participants in the nursing situation to study, interpret, and attest the nature and meaning of the lived events. The knowledge generated in phenomenological research is communicated in a manner that allows understanding, while protecting distinct individuals and groups.

The tools of this method are words and conceptualized ideas. The method is outlined in five phases:

1. Preparation of the nurse knower for coming to know. This entails confronting fear of openness, ambivalence, angular view, and being open to the angular views in the data.

2. Nurse knowing the other intuitively. This refers to the ability to "get into the rhythm and mobility of the other."

3. Nurse knowing the other scientifically. This is I-It relating and entails an analytic process. Relationships considered between components, trends, and patterns are conceptualized, and a sequential view of this experience is symbolically interpreted.

4. Nurse complementarily synthesizing known others. This phase involves comparing and synthesizing multiple known realities. An expanded view of the concepts is arrived at by this fourth phase.

5. Succession within the nurse from the many to the paradoxical one. The angular view is corrected and expanded. In this phase, nursing knowledge is moved forward (Paterson and Zderad, p 76-77, 1976).

This method has been used with groups of nurses to help them identify and describe those concepts they consider important in their own clinical nurse practice. The phenomenological method is being used in research by a number of nurse investigators.

Paterson and Zderad state that they do not believe their theory has been used as a basis for research (Paterson and Zderad, 1981). Paterson describes how she used Nursology to develop the concepts *comfort, clinical process,* and *all-at-once.* These concepts were identified by Paterson as fundamental to her own clinical practice (Paterson and Zderad, 1976; Paterson and Zderad, 1981).

Although the theory has probably not been used to date as a basis for nursing research, there is potential for doing so. As the concepts are further described and more precisely defined, propositional statements and hypotheses will be possible and empirical testing can be considered. As this is accomplished, the complementary relationship between phenomenology and empirical science will be more clearly shown.

Relationship to Nursing Education

The humanistic nursing model has been used by Paterson and Zderad as the theoretical base for classes with graduate psychiatric nursing students, a sixteen-week inservice class at the Veterans Administration Hospital in Northport, New York, and two-day seminars for practicing nurses throughout the country.

Documentation of its use in designing undergraduate curricula or graduate courses by other nursing educators does not appear in the literature. Content for inclusion in an undergraduate nursing curriculum is indirectly suggested in the theorists' writings. The existential framework necessitates a knowledge of philosophy, especially existential philosophy. Paterson and Zderad emphasize the relationship between nursing and art. Nurses may study the arts and the humanities to enrich their understanding of the human experience, may express their nursing worlds through various art forms, and may use the arts therapeutically (Paterson and Zderad, p 98, 1976). This suggests that history and literature may be as important as the more traditional psychology and sociology content of nursing curricula. Humanistic Nursing Theory's focus on nurse-patient relating provides rationale for including courses that emphasize modes of communication. The need for knowledge of family and growth and development theories is supported by Paterson and Zderad's beliefs that a person's present and future are affected by past experiences and that nursing varies with the amount, duration, and type of help required by the patient. Courses incorporating methods that assist values clarification and knowing of the self would be prerequisite to the nurse identifying his/her own angular view and being open to others. Recognition of person as a being relating to the world through the body implies that physical and biological science content would be included. That nursing varies with the diagnosis or disability of the patient supports inclusion of pathophysiology in a basic curriculum. Acquisition of technical skills and the ability to use technology in the care of incarnate man's physical needs are also suggested. Research is an inherent component of humanistic nursing. Nursology and positivistic science methodology would therefore be included. The theorists' existential valuing of each human being's capacity to become and their stated belief in the ability of each nurse to describe lived nursing experiences suggests use of the dialectical dialogue as the teaching-learning method of choice.

The theory's terminology is that of existential philosophy rather than nursing. The focus is in the processes of nurse-patient relating; clinical examples are primarily from mental health nursing situations. Despite these limitations it appears possible to develop a conceptual framework and an outline of content for an undergraduate curriculum. Development of specific course content, objectives, clinical experiences, and behavioral outcome criteria for evaluation would be much more difficult.

Relationship to Professional Nursing Practice

According to the theorists' own description of clinical situations, the theory has proven useful to them and other nurses in their practice, irrespective of clinical setting or speciality. Objective criteria for improvement in quality of patient care have not been identified. Rather, the individual nurse's judgment that care has improved and the improvement in the nurse's well-being are offered as support for its effectiveness. This is consistent with phenomenology's emphasis on individual meaning.

Paterson and Zderad do not ignore the need for the nurse at times to focus on some aspects of the patient's body or behavior. They point out that the body is a part of the whole person, and behavior is an expression of the person's mode of existence. While acknowledging that focusing on the whole person is necessary, it is still regarded as inhibiting true dialogical presence for the nurse. This bounded legitimization of concern for attention to physical status gives support for application of the theory in clinical nursing situations other than psychiatric mental health.

The difficulty of continuous "active presence" with the whole of the nurse's being is addressed by the theorists. In actual practice humanistic nursing may occur in various degrees and is viewed as a goal for which to strive or a value-shaping practice.

A theory of nursing which emphasized conscious decision-making and active involvement of the whole person in calling and responding would appear to have limited applicability in situations in which the nurse as helper interacts with a child or comatose patient. Paterson and Zderad use a quote from Buber to respond that the art of nursing can exist even if the relationship is not mutual:

"Even if the man to whom I say, Thou is not aware of it in the midst of his experience, yet relation may exist. For Thou is more than it realizes. No deception penetrates here: here is the cradle of the Real Life." (Buber, p 9, 1958)

It would be difficult for an inexperienced practitioner to move from reading about the theory to implementation and confidence that she/he was indeed practicing humanistic nursing. The existential influence on terminology (I-Thou, I-It, all-at-once, noetically transcending), emphasis on intuitive knowing, their belief that our limited language inhibits adequate description of the subjective and intersubjective aspects of relating makes operationalization difficult. Practitioners would be restrained by the need to answer such questions as: How do I give myself and receive back the other? How do I noetically transcend in relating to I-It? What criteria do I use when I analyze, classify, compare, and contrast? Answering these questions will require a sophisticated experiential and knowledge base.

SUMMARY

The humanistic nursing model, developed by Paterson and Zderad, is variously defined by the theorists as a nursing practice theory, a framework or approach to theory development, and as a metatheory. The purpose of the theory is to help nurses refine direct nursing care, advance nursing practice, and further nursing as a profession (Paterson, 1978). The method is phenomenological, a study of the nursing act itself. Paterson and Zderad's view of man and of philosophical inquiry is heavily influenced by existential philosophy. The theory is at a descriptive level. Paterson and Zderad are continuing the process of further description and conceptualization.

Humanistic Nursing Theory viewed as a model is significant as a philosophical perspective to guide nursing practice. The model viewed as a "framework or approach" is significant in guiding nurses in their own clinical theorizing to help them experience the intersubjective relating between them and their patients, reflect on these experiences, and then describe these experiences. The model viewed as a "metatheory" perhaps is the most accurate view of Humanistic Nursing Theory as presented by Paterson and Zderad. The model is abstract and open theoretically. Yet it is sufficiently abstract and open that theory can be derived from it.

The model is a highly significant contribution to nursing and appropriately takes its place alongside other nursing conceptual frameworks.

REFERENCES

Buber M: I and Thou, 2nd ed (trans. Ronald Gregor Smith). Charles Scribner's Sons, New York, 1958

Dewey J: The Knowing and the Known. Beacon Press, Boston, Massachusetts, 1949

Dickoff J, James P: A theory of theories: A position paper. Nursing Research, Vol 17, No 3, pp 197-203, 1968

Ellis R: Characteristics of significant theories. Nursing Research, Vol 17, No 3, pp 217-222, 1968

Farber M: The Aims of Phenomenology: The Motives, Methods, and Impact of Husserl's Thought. Harper & Row Publishers, Inc., New York, 1966

Hardy ME: Theories: Components, development, evaluation. Nursing Research, Vol 23, No 2, pp 100-106, 1974

Laing RD: The Politics of Experience. Ballantine Books Inc., New York, 1967

Maslow AH: The Psychology of Science. Henry Regnery Co., Chicago, Illinois, 1966

Natanson M: Phenomenology and the social sciences. In Vol 1, Northwestern University Press, Evanston, Illinois, 1973

Newman M: Theory Development in Nursing. F.A. Davis Co., Philadelphia, Pennsylvania, 1979

Parse RR: Man-Living-Health: A Theory of Nursing. John Wiley & Sons, New York, 1981

Paterson JG: The tortuous way toward nursing theory. In Theory Development: What, Why, How? National League for Nursing, New York, 1978

Paterson JG, Zderad LT: Humanistic Nursing. John Wiley & Sons, Inc., New York, 1976

Paterson JG, Zderad LT: Personal communication, October 1981

Reynolds PD: A Primer in Theory Construction. Bobbs-Merrill Co., Inc., Publishing, Indianapolis, Indiana, 1971

Rogers ME: An introduction to the theoretical basis of nursing, F.A. Davis Co., Philadelphia, Pennsylvania, 1970

Stewart D, Mickunas A: Exploring Phenomenology: A Guide to the Field and Its Literature. American Library Association, Chicago, Illinois, 1974

Strasser S: Phenomenology and the Human Sciences: A Contribution to
a New Scientific Ideal. Duquesne University Press, Pittsburgh, Pennsylvania, 1963

Warshay LH: The Current State of Sociological Theory: A Critical Interpretation. David McKay Co., Inc., New York, 1975

Zderad LT: From here-and-now to theory: Reflections on "how." In
Theory Development: What, Why, How? National League for Nursing, New York, 1978

Zderad LT: Personal communication, April 1982

Zeitlin TM: Rethinking Sociology: A Critique of Contemporary Theory.
Prentice-Hall, Inc., Englewood Cliffs, New Jersey, 1973

12

THE BETTY NEUMAN
HEALTH CARE SYSTEM MODEL

Ann L. Whall

INTRODUCTION

According to several of the major methods for classifying theoretical statements, as discussed in the introductory chapter, Neuman's Health Care System Model (1972, 1980) clearly fits into the category of that of model. In her model, Neuman focuses upon two major components, the nature of the relationship between the nurse and the patient, as well as the patient's response to stressors. In Neuman's view, the "patient" may be an individual, a group such as a family, or a community. Although hypotheses and principles might be developed from the model after explication and verification of concepts and propositions, this is not Neuman's primary purpose. Rather, for Neuman, the model is an attempt to provide a systems framework which will guide the actions of the professional care giver, i.e., assessment and intervention with patients. Thus the model is intended for use by various health care professionals.

Neuman's model is descriptive of a process which might be used by any health care professional (see Figure 12.1 for depiction of the model). That is, the process of assessing, intervening, and evaluating "a patient and his/her stressors" is when the two components identified above are considered the major focus of the

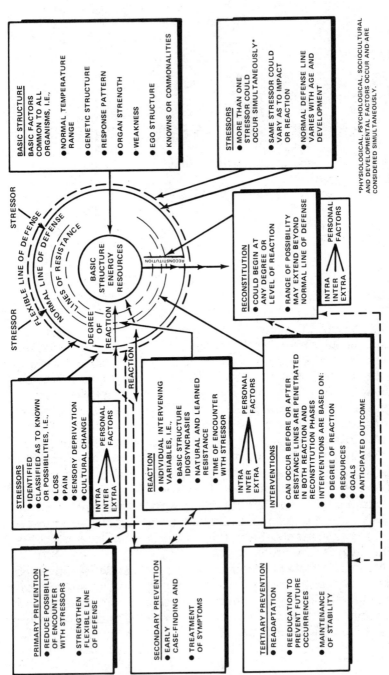

Figure 12.1. The Neuman Model. (*From:* Neuman B: A model for teaching total person approach to patient problems. Nursing Research, Vol 21, No 3, p 265, 1972. With permission of Betty Neuman. Published by American Journal of Nursing Co, New York)

model. The goal of the model in terms of health state does not receive as much emphasis as does the overall process which the professional caregiver employs. However, the ultimate goal of primary prevention and/or reconstitution is certainly implicit in the model. Neuman's model is reminiscent of the emphasis upon prevention of disease which was prevalent in the public health writings of the 1950s and 1960s (Hanlon, 1964). That is, the terms "levels of prevention" as well as "lines of defense" were often discussed in these sources.

In a conversation with Neuman, however, she stated that public health and/or community health influences were not consciously a part of her reasoning when she developed the model (Neuman, 1981). Rather, Neuman originally developed the model for educational purposes. The nursing program with which she was associated at the time wanted to examine conceptual frameworks which might be used to guide the curriculum. It was this impetus that motivated Neuman to develop the model. She conceptualized a way of approaching the health care of individuals, groups of individuals, and communities and visualized that different health care professionals would be interested in different variables as each utilized the model. Neuman thus developed the model to help others conceptualize a systems approach to health care. She believes that the work of the theorist is to challenge others to more fully develop a given model, thus, those who utilize the model might develop it more fully (Neuman, 1981).

Neuman states that her model provides a process for approaching varied nursing problems and for understanding the basic phenomena of interest—persons and their environment (p 121, 1980). The way in which the basic phenomena is conceptualized is that of a "patient" reacting to, or potentially reacting to, various stressors. A major value of this model appears to be conceptualizing the process by which a member of the health care system may relate to an individual, a group, or a community, and the way in which a multiplicity of data may be organized. In Neuman's view, nursing is concerned with *all* potential stressors; therefore, the way in which all the data regarding stressors and reaction to stressors may be organized is very important. The model itself does not specifically address ways in which intervention might be carried out; this is consistent with the purpose of the theorist, i.e., health care professionals in general and nursing in particular are challenged to further explicate the model.

BASIC CONSIDERATIONS

There are four basic concepts which have been identified as being present, either explicitly or implicitly, in all nursing models. These concepts are person, environment, health, and nursing. In addition, each nursing model presents other concepts which are specific to the model and which are used to explain the relationship of the four basic concepts. Neuman's model can be said to be a nursing model, even though it was designed for nursing as well as other health professionals, because the model addresses nursing, person, health, and environment.

Nursing and Nursing Activity

Neuman states that nursing is concerned with the total person and is a "unique" profession concerned with *all* the variables affecting an individual's response to stressors (p 121, 1980). The uniqueness of nursing is related to the number of totality of the variables with which nursing is concerned, and Neuman, in effect, states this. That is, nursing is concerned with a particular set of variables which stresses the patient. Neuman also states, however, that the model is appropriate for use with other health care providers but consistent with her viewpoint on the role of the theorist; she does not address how each health care provider would use the model differently (p 119, 1980). Neuman (1981) has stated that she purposefully used one model for all health care professions so that nursing might have a common language with other professions. Neuman also believes that nursing, with its broad perspective, should be in charge of coordinating health care.

The nurse in Neuman's model is seen as the "actor" or intervener who attempts to reduce an individual's encounter with certain stressors or attempts to mitigate the effect of certain stressors (p 124, 1980). In addition the nurse may intervene by strengthening the individual's ability to respond to the stressor. It appears from this brief description that a stressor in most cases is seen as potentially noxious, and that the nurse is an active participant in building the patient's defenses or in helping him/her to respond appropriately.

The patient is active in the sense that the meaning of an experience to the patient must be assessed (p 126, 1980). In addition, collaborative and progressive goal setting are terms used by Neuman to describe the activity between the nurse and the patient. Neuman states that once a major problem has been defined and classified, a decision must be made as to what form of intervention should take priority (p 129, 1980). In terms of who makes the decision, it appears consistent with the model that this is a collaborative decision with the nurse having a good deal of influence. Because the term patient is used rather than some other term, it would seem that the person is in a somewhat dependent or perhaps vulnerable state because of some illness or some other condition and thus in need of assistance from the health care system.

The nurse assists the patient quite differently depending upon the particular situation in terms of primary prevention, secondary prevention, or tertiary prevention. In each phase the nurse assesses differently and intervenes differently. For example, if the stressor is present in the patient's environment but has not broken through the normal line of defense (the primary level prevention level), then the nurse might assess the risk and seek to perhaps teach or assist the patient accordingly. If the stressor has penetrated the normal line of defense (the secondary level prevention level), then the nurse might act to determine the nature of any disease process and begin to deal with maladaptive processes. If the stressor has resulted in residual symptoms (the tertiary level prevention level), then the nurse may attempt to limit the effects perhaps by use of rehabilitative resources.

In summary, the nurse and/or other health care professional in the Neuman model is an active evaluator and intervener. The patient is seen as active but appears less so than the nurse due to some altered state. Nursing is described as unique and the uniqueness is related to the holistic nature as well as the number of the variables with which nursing is concerned. The nurse assesses all factors influencing the patient's perceptual field (p 125, 1980). Neuman states that, therefore, the professional caregiver's perceptual field must also be assessed because perception obviously influences the caregiver's actions. This self-assessment is interpreted to mean that the nurse examines his/her own biases, needs, and values before making care decisions. In a situation where the nurse or other caregiver appears to be most active, it seems essential that self-assessment be included.

Person

Person, or man in Neuman's terminology, is in some state of wellness and/or illness and is a dynamic composite of interrelationships between physiologic, psychologic, sociocultural, and developmental factors (p 121, 1980). Neuman further proposes that the total person must be viewed; the wholeness concept she states is related to the interrelationship of variables which determines the amount of resistance an individual has to any given stressor. Although this statement is not more fully explained, it tends to emphasize the dynamic character of the parts which influences the total person. The "wholeness' or totality of the individual is important, but because the definition of person as a physiologic, psychologic, sociocultural, and developmental being might be interpreted as a focus on the parts. It is important to identify that the focus appears to be the whole person. A holistic approach to the individual is indicated by the assessment categories, for these are holistic in nature (p 126, 1980). That is, assessment data to be considered is, for example, perception and meaning of the total experience to the individual, the individual's overall coping patterns, and his/her life style habits.

As addressed above, the person is seen as engaged in varying amounts of activity with regard to stressors and in need of assistance in certain instances. When stressors occur, the individual may need more information or other assistance to overcome stressors. Motivation is considered an intervention which the nurse may need to foster in the individual. That is, if a person ignores their diabetic diet, for example, the nurse would attempt to motivate the client in this regard.

The person is seen as possessing a normal line of defense. That is, each individual over time has evolved a normal range of responses which are referred to as normal lines of defense (p 121, 1980). Neuman further states that an individual's normal line of defense is in a sense an equilibrium state. The individual also has evolved a flexible line of defense over time. This is a reaction system or potential which can be used against stressors, e.g., psychological defenses. When an individual's normal line of defense or equilibrium is upset (for example, through the death of a spouse), the individual's flexible line of defense or reaction system would attempt to mitigate this stressor. The flexible line of defense in this case might be the individual's ability (built up over a time) to dissociate emotions from events. In this case, the surviving spouse might be able to delay the grief reaction as he/she makes the necessary arrangements.

In addition, according to the model, each person has internal lines of resistance which attempt to return the person to normalcy or equilibrium. To continue the example above, after the funeral the full impact of death might be fully experienced by the survivor. Although equilibrium is now upset and the flexible line of defense is no longer adequate, the survivor might now attempt by some ongoing activity, perhaps immersing himself/herself in their career, to return his/her life to a state of normalcy and or equilibrium.

There are some terms and relationships within the model which need to be more fully developed. For example, within the model, the normal line of defense is well defined but the definitions of flexible line of defense and internal lines of resistance are less well defined and must essentially be inferred or perhaps developed. A point to be considered in further model development is that if a stressor is to be viewed as primarily a noxious event to be avoided, and mitigated with a return to equilibrium, then personal growth would appear to be problematic. For example, an educational experience many times is a stressful event for individuals, but avoidance of the event would result in little growth on the part of the individual. Although the model implies that overcoming the stressor might be to apply oneself to educational pursuits, this growth producing disequilibrium aspect needs to be further developed. Thus the model might allow for the nurse to help a new student to experience disequilibrium, but support and encourage the student to draw upon his/her flexible lines of defense such as past successful coping strategies. Finally, the use of the term patient might be interpreted to connote a disease orientation although this is not the case. Perhaps further development might consider the use of the term person or client or some explicit rationale for use of the term patient to overcome any disease implication; a change might also indicate a more active participation by a client.

Health

Health is defined in terms of model components. Thus, a person's health is a state of wellness or illness determined by the four variables—physiologic, psychologic, sociocultural, and developmental. Health, then, is relative and in a dynamic state of flux. Health for one individual may mean a reconstitution state—e.g., using a prosthesis after amputation.

Health in the model is for the most part inferred and appears to be in essence the steady state of equilibrium or, graphically, a steady normal line of defense. This normal line of defense defines the parameters of the health state. Health is what the individual has become over time; it implies being in a state of flux in terms of relative strength. In the past someone may have experienced an attack of influenza and thereby have antibodies readily available. These antibodies constitute the individual's flexible line of defense which protects the individual's steady state. In another example, an individual who has experienced a psychotic depression, although now reconstituted, may have a biological predisposition to the condition. His/her flexible line of defense would, in this example, be more permeable than other individuals and is thus potentially less healthy. Health for the individual, thus, depends upon his/her genetic constitution and past experience. The advantage of this type of definition of health is that it allows for individual differences, i.e., health is not a perfect state or some absolute standard. Thus, the best possible state of health varies between persons and within persons at any given time.

Environment

Neuman states that there are both internal and external environments; the person maintains varying degrees of harmony and balance between the internal and external environment (p 122, 1980). This conceptualization of environment is a strength of the model, because this conceptualization allows greater latitude. Intrapsychic states, for example, may be conceptualized. Since the nurse is concerned with the stressor and the individual's reaction to it, the nurse is concerned with both the patient's internal and external environment. In other words, the nurse might consider the person's feelings, emotions, and perceptions and how these are affecting the individual as well as physical illness related to a stressor. It seems that the emphasis here is upon the totality of forces that may disturb the normal line of defense.

Interrelationship of Basic Concepts

The nurse is seen as an active participant with the patient and as external to the client. The patient is seen imbedded in an external (to person) environment but with an internal component and possibly in need of assistance from a nurse. Exactly when and if nursing is needed and the decision regarding this needs to be more fully developed. Health is a dynamic state influenced over time and in which the individual seeks to maintain some form of equilibrium. Stressors can be internal or external to the person and the nature of the stressor needs to be evaluated by the health care professional. Thus, another strength of the model lies in the interrelationships among concepts. That is, through this model, one is able to conceptualize the individual as being in varying states of health, the environment as being both internal and external to the individual and in a state of flux, and the nurse as an assessor and intervener in the overall process. Although some of the concepts and relationships need to be more fully developed, the basic nursing concepts are present and do fit with one another in a logical fashion.

INTERNAL ANALYSIS

An assumption is often defined as a proposition which may be accepted without proof. There are several types of assumptions but those with the most relevance here are implicit and explicit assumptions. A few of the major explicit assumptions which Neuman identifies have been paraphrased below (pp 119-121, 1980).

1. Each person is a unique individual with a normal range of responses.
2. There are many types of stressors which may upset an individual's equilibrium (normal line of defense).
3. The nature of the stressors may affect the extent to which a person may use their flexible line of defense.
4. A person's normal range of responses are called the normal line of defense. The flexible line of defense is a reaction system to be used against stressors.
5. When the flexible line of defense cannot protect against a stressor, the stressor upsets the equilibrium of the person.
6. Each person's internal resistance lines attempt to return the individual to normal.
7. Wellness or illness is determined by a dynamic state of a person's physiologic, psychologic, sociocultural, and developmental states.

These assumptions carry out this basic element of the models, i.e., the individual in interaction with his/her environment. It appears that other health care professionals could infer from the model the way in which to intervene between the stressor and the patient in some specific way. For example, a physiotherapist might identify the stressors affecting the patient's musculature and or bones. The intervention would be directed by this knowledge.

Some implicit assumptions can be inferred. For example, the patient's individuality is to be valued and attempts to maintain the steady state or health is a prime consideration. The individual as well as health professions have a major responsibility for maintaining this health state. In addition, the health care professionals are able to assist persons attain and maintain health.

Although the community and families are referred to by Neuman, the assumptions refer only to the individual. Neuman has stated that although the assumptions were originally conceptualized in terms of the individual, she hopes that others will expand these to other systems (Neuman, 1981). To develop the assumptions for larger health care systems such as a community or family, these questions will need to be addressed: What are communities' or groups' normal and flexible lines of defense? How are families or groups to be assisted to maintain steady states? What is the nature of a family's and community's flexible lines of defense? All of these questions may be addressed from inferences made in the model at the present time. However, the assumptions for these larger systems need to be explicitly developed and carefully evaluated.

Other Components of the Model

The main concepts identified by Neuman in her diagram are stressors, lines of defense, levels of prevention, individual variables, basic structure, interventions, and reconstitution (p 120, 1980) (See Figure 12.1.). Purposeful interventions are aimed at the reduction of stress factors and adverse conditions which either affect or could affect optimal functioning of an individual. All of these terms and levels of these terms have been theoretically defined by Neuman. Stressor, for example, is anything with a potential to disturb an individual's equilibrium or normal line of defense (p 121, 1980). In this regard, Neuman quotes Selye's definition of a stressor as a tension-producing stimulus.

Normal line of defense is referred to both as an individual's equilibrium and also as a normal range of responses developed by the individual over time. In terms of further development of this concept, the range of responses developed by an individual over time might need to be addressed. For example, might this include development of psychotic behavior? If a goal is to maintain equilibrium, how would this development be addressed? The flexible line of defense is referred to as an accordion-like effect which protects an individual against a stressor. Neuman states that the interaction-adjustment process contains variables that make up the flexible line of defense. These variables may be described further as the model is utilized, or they might be the subject of research upon the model. The lines of resistance are defined as factors which attempt to stabilize and return an individual to his/her normal line of defense should a stressor break through (p 121, 1980).

In terms of the types of concepts employed by Neuman in her model, Dubin (1978) would consider most relational units. That is, a relational unit is a property characteristic of a thing that can be determined only by relation among properties (p 62, 1978). Thus, when a stressor and an individual come into contact, one may speak of lines of defense or levels of prevention. Relational units are properties, e.g., reconstitution, derived from interaction of two or more other properties (stressors, individuals, and lines of resistance). Dubin states that relational units sum up properties of things and that one should keep in mind that other aspects of the relationship must be ignored because of the summing nature of the units (Dubin, p 63-64, 1978).

The basic terms which nursing models use—person, environment, health and nursing—are essentially summative units, or terms that stand for an entire complex of a thing. As Dubin suggests, relational units may be used to build theory, but summative units are too broad and cannot be used in theory building efforts. Thus, Neuman's model is at a broad level of specificity, but has potential in terms of derivation of a specific theory. One problem with nursing models in general is that empirical indicators for the terms are not readily identifiable. An empirical indicator is some operation employed by a researcher to measure a unit (Dubin, p 182, 1978). If Neuman's terms are primarily relational (see above), then the "tests" used must (according to Dubin) measure either a combination of combined properties or the interaction of properties. Thus the "tests" for Neuman's model might address the amount of resistance available in the flexible line of defense and/or the disequilibrium which results from interaction between the normal line of defense and the stressor.

There are two criteria for empirical indicators which have been used (Dubin, p 183, 1978). These are operationalism and reliability. For operationalism one must be able to observe the "thing happening"—a specific case of flexible lines of defense in operation against stressor must be observed. Reliability in this regard refers in part to ability of different observers to measure the same thing again and again. As can be seen from this discussion of Neuman's model, the model in itself is valuable in terms of an overall approach. The potential for derivation of more specific theory from the model exists, but much development is needed.

Analysis of Consistency and Adequacy

Hill (1966) has suggested three tests for theory adequacy: abstractness, cumulation, and predictability. Neuman's Total Person Approach to Patient Problems does abstract the situation. Not tied to specific and thus limited situations, the model presents an overview in which many problems may be analyzed. The model is cumulative in that each component builds upon the other. Once man and the environment are defined, stressors can be identified. Neuman's model, however, as with all models, is not at the level of predictability. That is, until more of the terms are operationally defined and empirical indicators identified, one cannot adequately address predictability.

Hardy (1974) has discussed theory adequacy. She states in part that addressing theory adequacy is related to assessing if operational definitions can be developed and tested. The theoretical definition of normal line of defense as range of responses which have evolved over time can be operationally defined. One operational definition suggested above might be an equilibrium of the immune system. The proportion of types of white blood cells, for example, might be addressed. Hardy goes on to state that operational adequacy of a theory is considered in terms of whether the operational definition can be measured and how accurately these reflect the theoretical definitions. After operational definitions have been developed for each of Neuman's theoretical concepts, the adequacy of the operational definitions may be addressed.

Hardy also discusses generality, which is similar to Hill's discussion of level of abstraction. As discussed above, Neuman's model is at a high level of abstraction, e.g., she discusses lines of resistance which may apply to multiple types of situations. Contribution to understanding is another point to be considered in terms of adequacy (Hardy, 1974). Herein lies a major contribution of this model, for a different way of viewing individuals and groups is presented. The model also suggests potential new directions for assessing individuals and situations. The model is not developed to the level of predictability suggested for theory testing by Hardy, nor is it purported to do so. Because pragmatic adequacy has to do with ability to predict, control, and explain, the pragmatic adequacy of Neuman's model is as yet limited. That is, prediction and control cannot yet be addressed. The explanatory nature of the model, however, is good, as the model would appear to explain in part individual stressors and the person's or groups' reaction to stressors.

Consistency considerations have to do with internal and external events. Neuman's model is internally consistent in that the three types of stressors, the three levels of prevention, and the four individual variables are discussed at the onset and throughout the model. There is a truthfulness to reality; for example, most stressors can be fit into one of Neuman's categories.

In terms of internal consistency, the uniqueness of nursing is not immediately evident and needs to be considered by the reader. The model does describe the concepts and relationships at outset and this logic is carried throughout. For example, man was defined in terms of four variables at the outset and at completion these four variables were again assessed. One point not addressed above has to do with Neuman's view that the model perhaps does not conflict with existing nursing models but may encompass them. Because the model discusses stressors and reactions to stressors in a type of multicausal function, the model would, however, conflict with those that assume acausality such as that of Rogers (1980).

Relationship to Research, Practice, and Education

Because scientific knowledge is basically a system for description and explanation (Reynolds, 1971), elements within the scientific body of knowledge describe "things" and why "events" occur. As with most nursing models, the operational definitions and empirical indicators have not been fully developed, but the model can be used as a guide for conceptualization of research problems and issues. Neuman's model might also be used to further nursing's body of knowledge through research upon the model itself. For example, some of the items research might address are: identification of the qualities of any normal and flexible lines of defense; identification of any quality that stressors must have in order to be defined as "sufficient" to overcome the flexible line of defense; and, identification of the types and patterns or any individual flexible line of defense. According to Neuman (1981), there are several ongoing research efforts to explicate various portions of the model; results of this research should be available in the near future. Two such researchers are Ziegler and Hough (1981). Ziegler reports that she is currently conducting a study validating a taxonomy of nursing diagnosis generated from the model. From this nursing diagnosis study, common stressors associated with individuals, groups, and communities will be addressed. Hough and Ziegler have recently completed chapters in a forthcoming work by Neuman (1982).

Neal (1981) has discussed the application of the Neuman model in practice. She sees the model as giving guidance to the nursing process. The model may guide the parameters for the assessment phase; the nurse in this view is concerned with assessing the normal line of defense or coping mechanisms. The nurse also assesses the individual's internal resistance factors, or in Neal's (1981) view, the homeostasis qualities that allow the individual to resist stressors. Neal also has completed a chapter in Neuman's forthcoming work (1982).

The model has been applied to practice by Beitler, Tkachuck, and Aamodt (1980). In terms of mental health nursing, Beitler et al. discuss stressors as being handled in terms of primary, secondary, and tertiary prevention. The mental health nurses in their discussion, at the level of primary prevention might attempt to promote acceptance of life as being composed somewhat of frustrating events. On the secondary level, the nurse might attempt to assist the client to work through feelings. On the tertiary level, the nurse might work with the environmental supports to assist the client in a crisis.

It would seem that as in the example above, the model could be used to conceptualize community health nursing. If, for example, the community problem was the return of large numbers of deinstitutionalized mental patients to the community, then the primary prevention might be seen as community education as to the nature of the deinstitutionalized patients. The secondary level of prevention might be to assist the community to draw upon its coping skills to deal with some of the more troublesome aspects of the situation. Perhaps a neighborhood block club might designate people on certain blocks to assist with the problems that occur once a home is established in the neighborhood. The tertiary level of prevention in this regard would be working with problems once they occurred. Perhaps there is, for example, a confrontation between the residents and neighbors that needs to be addressed. In this regard the neighborhood block club, plus the home operators and resident representatives, might meet to work out approaches.

In terms of education, the model was originally designed as a curriculum guide (Neuman, 1972; 1981). There are several different ways in which the model could be used to guide education; Ziegler and Hough (1981) are examining one such application. One way might be for a baccalaureate program on the first and second levels to explore the four variables which describe person. Thus, physiology, psychology, and sociology would be studied. The person as a developing being would also be studied in terms of the physiological, sociological, and psychological aspects. At the third and fourth levels, larger systems might be studied, the family and community, for example. Possible impending stressors and examples of preventive approaches specific to each developmental level could be studied. There are certainly other ways in which the model might be implemented to guide education; these ways in part indicate the versatility of the model. Lebold and David (1980) describe another approach to baccalaureate nursing education utilizing the Neuman model.

Neuman and Wyatt (1980) discuss the model as a guide to education at the master's level. They describe a program whereby nurse administrators are prepared. The program, which has been used to guide a university nursing administration program, uses a systems perspective and addresses the management system, the role of the nurse practitioner within the system, and the functions that nurses would carry out within the system such as client education and research.

SUMMARY

Neuman has presented an interesting and valuable model for the structure of the relationship between individuals, groups, and the nurse, as well as other health care professionals. Neuman stated that the model is an attempt to provide a framework for viewing health care problems which would be useful to various health care providers. In addition she has stated that one question that should be asked of any model is: "Does it contribute to nursing?" (Neuman, 1981). It seems that she has accomplished the goals of providing a broad framework and of contributing to nursing. Ellis (1968) has discussed that characteristics of significant theories are scope, complexity, testability, generation of information, and usefulness. Although this model is not at the level of a theoretical structure, these characteristics are relevant, because nursing models, after more testing and explication, may be developed into theoretical structures.

According to Ellis (1968), a theory has scope if it covers and relates a number of concepts and provides a potential framework for ordering observations. As discussed throughout this chapter, Neuman's model has scope of a fairly high order. Complexity according to Ellis means that multiple variables or relationships are considered. This is certainly true of Neuman's model. Testability according to Ellis is not a requisite for significance of a theory for "testability can be sacrificed in our era in favor of scope, complexity and clinical usefulness" (Ellis, p 220, 1968). The direct testing of portions of Neuman's model is being addressed, and the model is judged to have adequate scope, complexity, and clinical usefulness. According to Ellis, these characteristics are important during this early phase of nursing theory development. Finally, the model may be said to generate new information in terms of ways in which to address patient problems. To this end the model is found to be useful.

REFERENCES

Beitler B, Tkachuck B, Aamodt D: The Neuman stress adaptation approach to education for nurse administrators. *In* Riehl J, Roy C (eds): Conceptual Models of Nursing Practice, Appleton-Century-Crofts, New York, 1980

Dubin R: Theory Building. The Free Press, New York, 1978

Ellis R: Characteristics of significant theories. Nursing Research, Vol 17, No 3, pp 217-222, 1968

Hanlon J: Principles of Public Health Administration. C.V. Mosby Co., St. Louis, Missouri, 1964

Hardy M: Theories: Components, development, evaluation. Nursing Research, Vol 23, No 2, pp 100-107, 1974

Hill R: Contemporary developments in family theory. Journal of Marriage & Family, Vol 28, pp 3-6, 1966

Lebold M, David L: A baccalaureate nursing curriculum based on the Neuman health systems model. *In* Riehl J, Roy C (eds): Conceptual Models for Nursing Practice, Appleton-Century-Crofts, New York, 1980

Neal M: Personal communication, November 13, 1981

Neal M: Nursing care plans and the Neuman model. *In* Neuman B (ed): The Neuman Systems Model, Appleton-Century-Crofts, New York, 1982 (in press)

Neuman B: The Betty Neuman model: A total person approach to viewing patient problems. Nursing Research, Vol 21, No 3, pp 264-269, 1972

Neuman B: The Betty Neuman health-care systems model: A total person approach to patient problems. *In* Riehl J, Roy C (eds): Conceptual Models for Nursing Practice, Appleton-Century-Crofts, New York, 1980

Neuman B: Personal communication, September 8, 1981

Neuman B (ed): The Neuman Systems Model. Appleton-Century-Crofts, New York, 1982 (in press)

Neuman B, Wyatt M: The Neuman stress/adaptation systems approach to education for nurse administrators. *In* Riehl J, Roy C (eds): Conceptual models for nursing practice, Appleton-Century-Crofts, New York, 1980

Reynolds P: A Primer in Theory Construction. Bobbs-Merrill Co., Inc., Indianapolis, Indiana, 1971

Rogers ME: A science of unitary man. *In* Riehl JP, Roy C (eds): Conceptual Models for Nursing Practice, 2nd ed, Appleton-Century-Crofts, New York, 1980

Ziegler S, Hough L: Personal communication, December 3, 1981

13

IMOGENE M. KING:
A THEORY FOR NURSING

Paula J. Gonot

INTRODUCTION

The development of Imogene King's ideas about nursing and science can be traced through her publications. In 1964, King referred to nursing as an art, a profession, and an occupation. She maintained, however, that the knowledge base for practice was in need of further organization. Four years later, King (1968) was refining her own conceptual frame of reference as a means of organizing the knowledge used by nurses in a meaningful fashion. The formal introduction of King's conceptual model of three interacting systems—personal, interpersonal, and social—came in *Toward a Theory for Nursing* (1971). In this text (1971), King speaks of nursing as a discipline and as an applied science with emphasis on the derivation of knowledge from other disciplines. She speculated that through systematic conceptualization the unknown domain of nursing theory will emerge as a science of human behavior. In the conclusion, however, King states that "nursing is not yet a science" (p 124, 1971). By 1978, in explaining the "why" of theory development, one notes a shift in King's views. She suggests that one must "think about nursing as a science and the relationship between theory and research as a way to build scientific knowledge" (p 11, 1978). There is also evidence that King has begun to reformulate her original conceptual framework, the result of which is her most recent publication—*A Theory for Nursing* (1981). Herein King makes reference to the systematic and theoretical approach to the professional practice of nursing, and encourages nurses to engage in the scientific endeavors of theory development and research. The emphasis clearly remains on the applied aspect of the discipline. "Nurses are expected to integrate knowledge from natural and behavioral sciences and to apply knowledge in concrete situations" (p 9, King, 1981). Further, King has delineated the previously "unknown" domain of nursing as including "promotion of health, maintenance and resotration of health, care of the sick and injured, and care of the dying" (p 4, 1981).

Comparing *Toward a Theory for Nursing* (1971) to *A Theory for Nursing* (1981) alerts the reader to a number of other changes in King's thinking which have evolved over the past decade. In the former text, through an extensive literature review combined with her own empirical observations, King induced four generalizations she believed to be universal to the discipline. These were social systems, health, perception, and interpersonal relations (pp 20-21, 1971). The definitional statements presented for these four concepts had foundations in various behavioral theories and terms, e.g., role, organization, communication, development, and were supported by multiple citations. Some of the terms used to elaborate the four major components of the 1971 text have been extrapolated and identified as substantive concepts in the 1981 text. In fact, the number of concepts in the 1971 model has been increased fourfold in the 1981 version.

In *A Theory for Nursing* (King, 1981), the concept of health is presented as an essential dimension of nursing and health care; yet is not identified as one of the major components of the open systems framework. There is less indication of a dichotomy, i.e., a health-illness continuum. Illness is more consistently referred to as an interference in the life cycle. The most significant change in the definition of health from 1971 to 1981 is the use of the word "adjustment" rather than "adaptation."

The latter change is in keeping with King's reformulations of person and environment, as well as their relationship. In 1971, King repeatedly characterized whole *man* (her term) as an additive composite: biologic/physical—psychologic/emotional—

social. Whereas similar terms have been used in the 1981 text when citing the works of other theorists and researchers, King suggests:

> It is the whole *person* interacting with the environment where one places artificial boundaries around a segment of that wholeness for the purpose of studying events in open systems (p 97, 1981). (Note: In the 1981 book, King did not use the term "man," instead she used terms such as "person", "human being", "individual.")

In 1971, King espoused the belief of man as an open system. However, man and environment were dichotomized, with the former reacting to the latter, as in a closed system. She spoke of energy exchange *within* and *external* to the human organism leading to behavioral responses (p 25, 1971). There was no mention of interaction/exchange *between* the two. Von Bertalanffy's concept of open systems extends beyond the stimulus-response formula and implies action, spontaneity, and undetermined boundaries (1969). Accordingly, King now addresses "a dynamic state of a human being which involves an exchange of energy and information between the person and the environment for regulation and control of stressors" (p 98, 1981). Only peripheral attention was given to the environment in the original model (1971). With King's reformulation of open systems, however, the environment is afforded substantial consideration throughout this new text (1981). These changes demonstrate King's refinement toward a "less closed" conceptualization of open system. Yet, there are still some inconsistencies with Von Bertalanffy's (1969) formulation of open system as reflected in King's use of terms such as "adjust," "conform," and "react," when referring to the person-environment relationship (pp 4-5, 19-20, 1981).

Finally, an integral thread of the conceptual framework as introduced in 1971 was the nursing process. In the 1981 text, King presents a theory of goal attainment which she has deduced from her revised model. It seems that the latter theory represents, in essence, an elaboration and refinement of King's formulation of the nursing process. Henceforth, the discussion and analysis will pertain to King's conceptual model as set forth in *A Theory for Nursing* (1981).

ANALYSIS OF BASIC CONSIDERATIONS

Person

Human beings are viewed as open systems interacting with the environment, each exhibiting permeable boundaries permitting an exchange of matter, energy, and information (King, p 69, 1981). Within the conceptual framework of three dynamic interacting systems, individuals are called personal systems. When individuals form groups they are called interpersonal systems. Social systems are created when groups with common interests and goals come together within a community or society (King, pp 10-11, 1981). The interrelationship of these systems is schematically diagrammed in Figure 13.1.

Each human being is conceptualized as a unique total system, the care of whom is the focus of nursing. King has explicated her philosophical assumptions about human beings as follows: individuals are social beings; sentient beings; rational beings; reacting beings; perceiving beings; controlling beings; purposeful beings; action-oriented beings; and, time-oriented beings. Individuals have rights as well as responsibilities (p 143, 1981).

In the process of human interactions, individuals react to persons, events, and objects in the environment in terms of their perceptions, expectations, needs, values, and goals. King identifies six concepts as relevant to understanding human beings as persons: 1) perception; 2) self; 3) body image; 4) growth and development; 5) time; and, 6) space (pp 19-20, 1981). These concepts are described and defined with personal systems, and are reviewed in a subsequent section of this chapter.

Environment

The environment is also conceptualized as an open system exhibiting permeable boundaries permitting an exchange of matter, energy, and information with human beings (King, p 69, 1981). King proposes that an understanding of the ways human beings interact with their environment to maintain health is essential to nurses (p 2, 1981). Reference is made to both the internal and external environment of human beings. "The internal environment of human beings transforms energy to enable them to adjust to continuous external environmental changes." Satisfaction in the performance of daily living depends

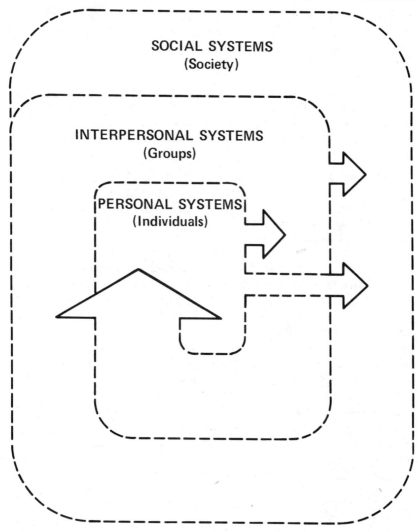

Figure 13.1. A Conceptual Framework for Nursing: Dynamic Interacting Systems. (*From:* King IM: Toward a Theory for Nursing. John Wiley & Sons, Inc., New York, p 11, 1981. With permission of I. M. King and John Wiley & Sons, Inc.)

upon harmony and balance in each person's environment (King, pp 4-5, 1981).

The implication here is not that the environment is an immovable force to which human beings must conform. Practice situations are cited, for example, where nurses must assess the environment and make alterations conducive to promoting health. Further, King states that "the moving forces in nursing are imbedded in the dynamics of society in which the process of change alters the environment" (p 11, 1981).

Health

Health is espoused as "a high priority in the hierarchy of values in society." It is a process of growth and development that is not always smooth and without conflict (King, p 4, 1981). King defines health as:

> Dynamic life experiences of a human being, which implies continuous adjustment to stressors in the internal and external environment through optimum use of one's resources to achieve maximum potential for daily living (p 5, 1981).

Whereas health is viewed as a functional state in the life cycle, illness indicates an interference in the cycle. Drawing upon her earlier work (1971), King relates health to the way individuals deal with the stresses of growth and development while functioning within the cultural pattern in which they were born and to which they attempt to conform (pp 4-5, 1981). Health is elsewhere more simply characterized as the ability to function in social roles (King, p 143, 1981). As noted in the introduction, the domain of nursing involves the promotion, maintenance, and restoration of health as well as care of the sick, injured, and dying.

Nursing

The goal of nursing "is to help individuals maintain their health so they can function in their roles" (King, pp 4-5, 1981). The universally accepted human service intent of practice is clear. King defines nursing as:

> A process of human interactions between nurse and client whereby each perceives the other and the situation; and through communication, they set goals, explore means, and agree on means to achieve goals (p 144, 1981).

The essential variables in nursing situations are identified as follows:

1. Geographical place of the transacting system, such as the hospital;

2. Perceptions of nurse and patient;
3. Communications of nurse and patient;
4. Expectations of nurse and patient;
5. Mutual goals of nurse and patient; and,
6. Nurse and patient as a system of interdependent roles in a nursing situation (King, p 88, 1981).

The quality of nurse-patient interactions may have a positive or negative influence on the promotion of health in any nursing situation (King, 1981).

It is within this interpersonal system of nurse-client that the traditional steps of the nursing process are carried out. "The interpretation of specific information (assessment) to plan, implement, and evaluate nursing care is the function of the professional nurse" (King, p 9, 1981). The same diagram (Figure 13.2) used to depict a process of interaction in both the conceptual framework (p 61, 1981) and the theory of goal attainment (p 145, 1981) was presented in King's 1971 text as a method of studying nursing process.

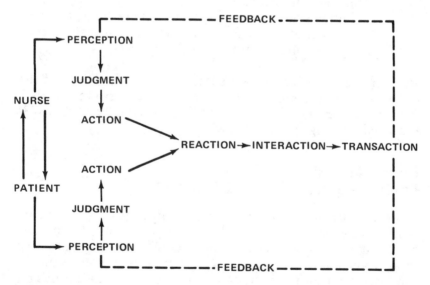

Figure 13.2. A Process of Human Interactions. (*From:* King IM: Toward a Theory for Nursing. John Wiley & Sons, Inc., New York, p 61, 1981. With permission of I. M. King and John Wiley & Sons, Inc.)

By way of explanation: nurse and patient meet in some situation, perceive each other, make judgments about the other, take some mental action, and react to each one's perceptions of the other. Since these behaviors cannot be directly observed, one can only make inferences about the same. The next step in the process is interaction which can be directly observed. Determination of the last term in the diagram, i.e. transaction, is dependent upon the achievement of a goal (King, pp 60-61, 1981).

Specific assumptions about nurse-client interactions made explicit by King are cited now because they are relevant to the nursing process:

1. Perception of nurse and of client influence the interaction process.
2. Goals, needs, and values of nurse and client influence the interaction process.
3. Individuals have a right to knowledge about themselves.
4. Individuals have a right to participate in decisions that influence their life, their health, and community services.
5. Health professionals have a responsibility to share information that helps individuals make informed decisions about their health care.
6. Individuals have a right to accept or to reject health care.
7. Goals of health professionals and goals of recipients of health care may be incongruent (pp 143-144, 1981).

Some of these philosophical assumptions are derivations of the values of organized professional nursing as set forth in the ANA *Code for Nurses* (1976) and *Standards for Nursing Practice* (1973) and cited by King (pp 11-12, 1981).

Interrelationships of Person, Environment, Health, and Nursing

Many aspects of the interrelationships between these concepts have been described in the above paragraphs. Person and environment are open systems continuously exchanging matter, energy, and information. This interaction may or may not be conducive to health promotion and, as such, has implications for the practice of professional nursing. The interrelationship is summarized in an overall assumption upon which the conceptual framework and the theory of goal attainment are based: "The focus of nursing is human beings interacting with their environment leading to a state of health for individuals, which is an ability to function in social roles" (King, p 145, 1981).

INTERNAL ANALYSIS OF THE MODEL

Before analyzing King's model, the three interacting systems of which the conceptual framework is comprised must be placed in perspective. From a systems approach, each entity is simultaneously a part and a whole. Any unit is made up of parts to which it is a whole, the suprasystem; and, at the same time, is part of some larger whole of which it is a component, or subsystem. The systems approach requires the designation of a "focal" system which is the system of primary attention. One then addresses the component parts (the subsystems) of that focal system, as well as the significant environment (the suprasystems) of which the focal system is a part, or to which it is related (Anderson and Carter, pp 8-9, 1974).

One can easily conclude that the interpersonal system is the focal system of King's conceptual framework. The primary attention afforded interpersonal systems is evidenced by:

1. The relatively greater detail provided the description of concepts within this system
2. The fact that the theory of goal attainment was derived mainly from component concepts of the interpersonal system
3. The theory of goal attainment describes the interpersonal system of nurse-client
4. King's reference to the conceptual framework of *inter-personal* systems rather than to that of *interacting* systems (p 144, 1981).

Personal systems, i.e., individuals, are the components or subsystems of interpersonal systems. Social systems designate the various environments or suprasystems in which interpersonal systems are experienced. The concepts identified in both personal and social systems serve to enhance one's understanding of interpersonal systems. It is, therefore, not surprising that of the sixteen concepts presented in the model, those most pertinent to interpersonal systems and the theory of goal attainment are developed more extensively in the text. Consequently, the components of the model will be analyzed and evaluated in accord with King's differential presentation of each.

Prior to analyzing the model's components, the basic assumptions and values inherent in the conceptualizations must be considered. The extent to which these are recognized and made explicit will be evaluated. As noted earlier, philosophical assumptions and values basic to personal systems, interpersonal systems, nursing process and practice, and the theory of goal attainment were clearly explicated by King (pp 12, 143-144, 1981). Further, these are viewed as being consistent with the definitions of concepts as well as the relationships proposed between them. This is not the case, however, with social systems. Herein, various statements reflect implicit assumptions and generalizations drawn by King.

The concepts presented as substantive content for nursing in each of the three interacting systems of the framework are as follows (King, pp xi-xii, 1981).

Personal	Interpersonal	Social
Perception	Human Interactions	Organization
Self	Communication	Authority
Growth and	Transactions	Power
Development	Role	Status
Body Image	Stress	Decision Making
Space		
Time		

In order to identify these concepts as types of theory building units, Dubin's (1969) classification system is used. A brief description of four unit types will be offered, and the concepts will be classified according to how King has conceptualized each.

The enumerative unit is universal; the characteristic property is always present, in all the states (conditions) under which the thing can be found. Any unit for which there is a zero value or an absent condition is not an enumerative unit (Dubin, pp 58-60, 1969). Those concepts which constitute enumerative units are perception, growth and development (as measured by age), space, time, communication, role, and stress. Note that communication is included here because "one cannot not communicate" (Satir, 1967; Watzlawick, et. al., 1971).

An associative unit describes a property characteristic of a thing, the value of which may be zero or negative, or both, in one or more states (Dubin, pp 60-62, 1969). Authority, power, status, and decision-making are associative units.

A relational unit is defined as a property characteristic of a thing that can be determined only by relation among properties. This relation is based either on interaction among properties or on the combination of properties. It represents a property of two or more properties of things; both properties and things can be plural (Dubin, pp 62-63, 1969). Self, body image, human inter-actions, transactions, and organization are relational units.

The summative unit is a global unit that stands for an entire complex thing. It draws together a number of different properties of a thing and gives them a label that highlights one of the more important properties (Dubin, pp 66-68, 1969). Personal, inter-personal, and social systems each represent a summative unit.

Dubin points out that it is possible that a unit employed in a theory may satisfy the definition of two or more classes of units at the same time. This fact is not necessarily problematic, but serves to alert the theorist that the same unit may be used differently within various models (pp 68-69, 1969). An example of such a unit is growth and development. When age is used as the measure of growth and development, the enumerative unit is appropriate. Yet, if one considers the theoretical complexity of the process of growth and development, classification as a relational unit is more fitting.

Personal Systems

King asserts that following a literature review in nursing and related fields whereby characteristics of concepts are identified, an operational definition is formulated, and application to nurs-ing situations is presented (p 23, 1981). This format is basically adhered to throughout the text with the exception of an opera-tional definition. More often, one finds a theoretical definition which gives meaning to the term in context of the model. Further, the concepts vary in generality within and between the three interacting systems (Hardy, 1974).

Perception is presented as a basic concept in both the framework and the theory of goal attainment, and is a major component in the process of human interactions. It is defined as:

> A process of organizing, interpreting, and transforming information from sense data and memory; a process of human transactions with environment; gives meaning to one's experience, represents one's image of reality, and influences one's behavior (King, p 24, 1981).

Growth and development describe the processes that take place in individuals' lives to help them move from potential for achievement to self-actualization. Age is a critical variable in any nursing situation because it defines the stage of each person's developmental tasks and their responses to each other. The concept of growth and development is another component in the theory of goal attainment (King, p 31, 1981).

Reviewing definitions of the other four concepts in light of the above definitions and interrelationships within personal systems can lead one to identification of a series of self-correlation among concepts. To illustrate: perception is a basis for developing a concept of self which is reflected in patterns of growth and development; knowledge of self and growth and development helps one understand body image; body image is an integral component of growth and development which, in turn, influences a concept of self. Spatial-temporal dimensions of the environment are presented as influencing perceptions, self, body image, and growth and development (King, pp 24-47, 1981). Quoting King, "if this sounds circular, it is, because they are facets of human experience" (p 142, 1981). Nevertheless, the relationships between these concepts fail to meet the criteria of logical adequacy (Hardy, 1974). As far as the semantics, or the meanings attributed to concepts, however, these are similar to meanings used by other scholars (Reynolds, 1971). Further, the terminology can be used meaningfully with, or applied to, phenomena observed in nursing (Ellis, 1968).

Interpersonal Systems

As suggested earlier, this system is the major focus of the framework as well as the basis for derivation of a theory for goal attainment. Each of the concepts within this system is used in developing the latter theory. The process of human interactions was schematically depicted and explained earlier in this chapter. Perception, communication, and transactions are the major concepts presented as fundamental for understanding human interactions as interpersonal systems. One communicates on the basis of perceptions with persons and things in the environment. Accuracy of perception increases effectiveness of one's actions. Effectiveness in interactions cannot be understood without considering the variable of purpose or goal (King, pp 80-82, 1981). The informational component of interactions can be observed as communication. The valuational component of interactions can be observed as transaction "because one obviously values a goal, identifies means to achieve it, and takes action to attain it" (King, pp 61-62, 1981).

"Communication is the structure of significant signs and symbols that brings order and meaning to human interaction"

(King, p 62, 1981). It is one form of the process whereby matter, energy, and information is exchanged. Some universal character-istics of communication are verbal, nonverbal, situational, per-ceptual, transactional, and irreversible. All human activities that link person to person and person to environment are forms of communication (King, pp 69, 79, 1981).

Whereas communication is the transfer of information between two or more individuals, transaction is the transfer of value between two or more persons. Both kinds of interaction are necessary. Transactions are "a process of interaction in which human beings communicate with the environment to achieve goals that are valued." Transactions are goal-directed behaviors which, when made, reduce tension or stress in a situation (King, pp 81-82, 1981).

The concept of human interactions has been classified as a relational unit. The units of perception, communication, and transactions are conceptualized as being properties of human interactions. Consequently, more self-correlating relationships are evident. King seems to have been intent on the reader understanding human interactions as interpersonal systems. This being the case, the latter two components could have been reformulated as one unit. The presentation of human inter-actions as a major concept in the framework would have thereby been negated, thus avoiding the self-correlations and resultant logical inadequacy.

The remaining two concepts presented in the interpersonal systems are role and stress. King suggests that the concept of role is relevant to each of the three interacting systems in her framework. It is presented within interpersonal systems "because roles identify interactive relationships and modes of communica-tion" (p 85, 1981). Role is essential within personal systems since an individual's behavior is influenced by a concept of self, which includes one's perceptions, needs, and goals. The concept has relevance within social systems when considering expectations inherent in assuming a position in a formal organization (King, pp 91-93, 1981). From a synthesis of diverse definitions, three elements are identified as giving meaning to the concept of role:

1. Role is a set of behaviors expected when occupying a position in a social system;
2. Rules or procedures define rights and obligations in a position in an organization; and,

3. Role is a relationship with one or more individuals interacting in specific situations for a purpose (King, p 93, 1981).

Whenever one is enacting a role, there is a potential for conflict which may increase stress in the environment. King's definition of stress is:

A dynamic state whereby a human being interacts with the environment to maintain balance for growth, development, and performance, which involves an exchange of energy and information between the person and the environment for regulation and control of stressors (King, p 98, 1981).

Stressors are persons, objects, and/or events. Stress can be experienced as positive or negative, constructive or destructive.

The relationship between human interactions and role has the potential for self-correlation, depending upon the manner in which role is conceptualized. If, for example, role is defined as a relationship a preposition linking this concept with human interactions would be circular. Propositional statements relating the concept role or stress with communication, transactions, perception, or with each other would not likely prove logically inadequate.

An additional idea presented within interpersonal systems is that of reciprocally contingent interaction where the behavior of one person influences the behavior of the other. "To establish this kind of relationship participation is required by both individuals" (King, p 85, 1981).

Social Systems

This system has been perceived as the suprasystem in which interpersonal systems are experienced. The concepts presented herein—organization, authority, power, status, and decision making—serve to identify various factors which may impact upon human interactions. King suggests that there are social forces in constant motion in social systems; the interplay of these forces influences social behavior, interactions, perceptions, and health (p 113, 1981).

Organization is operationally defined as "composed of human beings with prescribed roles and positions who use resources to accomplish personal and organizational goals" (King, p 119,

1981). Authority is said to: 1) be legitimate and perceived by individuals; 2) reside in the position held by a person who distributes the sanctions and rewards; 3) reside in the competence of a person with special knowledge and skills, such as professionals; and, 4) reside in the person who uses human relation skills to exercise leadership in a group (King, p 124, 1981). Power is "the process whereby one or more persons influence other persons in a situation"; it defines a situation such that people will accept what is being done while they may not agree with it (King, p 127, 1981). Status is the position of an individual in a group or a group in relation to other groups in an organization (King, p 129, 1981). Decision making in organizations is "a dynamic and systematic process by which goal-directed choice of perceived alternatives is made and acted upon by individuals or groups to answer a question and attain a goal (King, p 132, 1981). These concepts are meaningfully defined in terms of conceptualizations offered by other scholars in the field. Though general propositional statements are made relating the concepts within social systems, the specificity required to assess for logical adequacy is lacking. Yet there are no apparent flaws in that which is presented.

In keeping with the format of the text, King discusses the implications of each social systems concept for nursing. It is within these discussions that implicit assumptions and generalizations are reflected wherein relevant contingencies may not have been taken into account.

Thus far, the meaning and logical adequacy of the three interacting systems has been evaluated. The assumptions and definitions of concepts within personal and interpersonal systems are valid. Yet the logical adequacy in these systems is limited by the identified self-correlating propositions. Though the definitional and general propositional statements presented within social systems are valid, the adequacy of some of the assumptions and generalizations are not substantiated. When assessing the internal consistency of the model, one must use care. In the literature reviews preceding the characteristics and definitions of each concept, a number of various definitions are offered as presented by other theorists. These definitions should not be confused with those developed by King. When these distinctions are made, it appears that King has employed the concepts in a rather consistent manner throughout the model.

Next, the empirical adequacy of the model can be evaluated. Operational definitions permit the validity of concepts to be assessed, as well as the empirical relevance of the conceptualizations (Hardy, 1974). The concepts which have been operationally defined are mainly those which have been utilized in the theory of goal attainment. These operational definitions accurately reflect the theoretical concepts (Hardy, 1974). From the operational definitions, both propositions and hypotheses have been derived within the theory.

Theory of Goal Attainment

The theory of goal attainment has been derived primarily from interpersonal systems. The concepts utilized are interactions, perception, communication, transaction, role, stress, and growth and development. The spatial-temporal dimensions of the immediate environment are also considered (King, p 145, 1981). A basic assumption in the theory is that generally patients and nurses communicate information, mutually set goals, and take action to attain goals (King, p 157, 1981).

The concepts as presented within the theory are congruent with their conceptualizations in the framework. The propositions deduced from the theory are also consistent with the relational statements previously set forth. The theory focuses on the human interaction of nurse-patient as experienced in the nursing situation. King also reports on the descriptive study which was conducted to test the theory. A major assumption of the study was that nurse and patient exhibit reciprocally contingent behavior whereby the behavior of one person influences the behavior of the other and vice versa (King, p 151, 1981). Prior to implementing this study, a series of observations resulted in an inductively derived operational definition of transaction (King, p 151-153, 1981). The operational definition, however, reflects more than the theoretical definition of transaction. All of the observable steps in the process of human interaction are encompassed, beginning at the point when one person initiates behavior toward the other. Following this activity, research was conducted to describe nurse-patient interactions that lead to transactions in concrete nursing situations. The design was intended to answer these questions:

1. What elements in nurse-patient interactions lead to transactions?
2. What are the relationships between the elements in the interactions that lead to transactions?

3. What are the essential variables in nurse-patient interactions that result in transactions (King, p 151, 1981)?

As was pointed out, the theory of goal attainment represents, in essence, an elaboration and refinement of King's formulation of the nursing process. As King suggests, testing the theory provides "empirical data about nursing process phenomena related to human interaction" (p 152, 1981). This is evidenced by the resultant classification system of nurse-patient interactions whereby elements in interactions are delineated as: action, reaction, disturbance (problem), mutual goal setting, exploring means to achieve goal, agreeing on means to achieve goal, and transaction—goal achieved (King, p 156, 1981).

Development of a classification system of nurse-patient interactions constitutes only the initial phase of testing the theory of goal attainment. Subsequent phases would involve designing studies whereby hypotheses generated by King, as well as by others, can be tested (p 155-156, 1981). As evidence which either supports or refutes the theory is accumulated, some conclusions about empirical adequacy can be reached (Hardy, 1974).

The theory of goal attainment is characterized by a relatively high degree of generality. The process of nurse-patient interaction is applicable to all age groups, to all nursing functions (i.e., promotion, maintenance, and restoration of health, and care of the sick, injured, and dying), and to all practice settings and specialty areas. Finally, in its current stage of development and testing, the theory affords description and explanation. Contingent upon research findings and further refinement, the pragmatic adequacy of the theory of goal attainment may be enhanced as the theory has the potential for predicting the outcomes/effectiveness of nurse-patient interactions (Hardy, 1974; King, 1981).

Final Internal Evaluation of the Model

To complete the internal evaluation, King's model will be critiqued using some of the characteristics of significant theories for nursing proposed by Ellis (1968). Scope refers to the number of concepts covered in the model, and reflects its potential for ordering observations about a variety of phenomena (Ellis, p 219, 1968). King's systems framework encompasses sixteen concepts, as well as formulations of person, environment, health, and

nursing practice. Of these concepts, at least six meet the definition of relational units characterized by a number of properties.
These facts attest to the breadth of King's model and, thus, its
potential significance for nursing. The theory of goal attainment
is just one of many theories which could be deduced from King's
framework. King suggests, for example, an interpersonal stress
theory and a control theory (p 143, 1981). Other avenues for
theory development include spatial-temporal perspectives, role
socialization, and organizational power, to name a few.

Closely related to scope is the complexity of the model, the
multiplicity of variables and relationships addressed (Ellis, 1968).
The sheer number of concepts presented in King's model contributes to its complexity. This complexity may account for the logical inadequacies noted in some of the propositions.

A prime characteristic for significance of theories is that of
usefulness for clinical practice. Significant theories must be
useful in developing and guiding practice (Ellis, 1968). The focal
system of interpersonal systems and the derived theory of goal
attainment which describes and explains nursing process are,
indeed, relevant to practice. To quote King:

> Some of the essential variables have been identified in
> the empirical description of the theory of goal attain-
> ment that provides knowledge of process and outcomes
> (goals attained). Process and outcomes are the heart of
> quality assurance programs in nursing (p 157, 1981).

As noted above, the theory also has potential for predicting and
controlling the effectiveness of nurse-patient interactions. King
has provided an additional contribution to practice in the 1981
text. She has modified the Problem Oriented Medical Record
(POMR: Weed, 1969) into a Goal Oriented Nursing Record
(GONR). The GONR is offered as a means to facilitate the application of the theory of goal attainment by nurses practicing in
health care systems (King, p 157, 1981). This underscores the
usefulness of the model and theory for clinical practice.

The final question to be answered is whether or not the
model generates new information. According to Ellis (1968),
theories which do not have any other characteristics of significance may be significant if they generate hypotheses. King has
derived and presents seven hypotheses from her theory (p 156,
1981). From the variety of other theories which could be deduced
from the model, the number of hypotheses seems unlimited. In

conclusion, significant theories for nursing are those which include the patient as an essential component (Ellis, 1968). King's model clearly meets this final criterion of significance.

EXTERNAL ANALYSIS OF THE MODEL

Relationship to Nursing Research

King's conceptual model (1981) has potential for invoking both inductive and deductive arguments through its refinement. Within the text, King presents the methodology for the first phase of testing the theory of goal attainment (pp 150-156, 1981). This descriptive study produced a classification system to analyze nurse-patient interactions. King suggests that future studies need to be designed to test hypotheses derived from the theory. The following is one example of such a hypothesis:

> Role conflict experienced by patients, nurses, or both, decreases transactions in nurse-patient interactions (King, p 156, 1981).

If this hypothesis were to be empirically substantiated, role conflict would be predictive of decreased transactions.

Hypotheses could be generated from propositional statements linking concepts among or between the three interacting systems. For example, relationships could be proposed and tested between the concepts of body image and space, self and role, stress and power, authority and status.

King states that if nurses are "to be effective in their professional roles they must have an understanding of the background of individuals in social systems and of health care systems within which they function" (p 135, 1981). The emphasis here is on knowledge for the practitioner. This model also has the potential for guiding research on social systems and the concepts defined therein which would be useful for nurse administrators, managers, and supervisors in their respective roles. The multifacets of King's conceptual framework affords the researcher a variety of avenues of inquiry into both basic and applied knowledge.

Relationship to Nursing Education

The establishment of programs within institutions of higher learning presupposes an identified branch of knowledge, i.e., a discipline. As Donaldson and Crowley explain, a discipline is characterized by a unique perspective, a distinct way of viewing phenomena, which ultimately defines the limits and nature of its inquiry. Consequently, there is a crucial need for identification of the structure of the discipline of nursing in our educational programs. The problem is not to devise this structure, but to make it explicit (pp 113-114, 1978). Nursing models explicate a framework for educational programs and give direction to research activities whereby theories of the middle range can be deduced which guide practice.

King gives a good deal of attention to the model's applicability to education. Her enthusiasm is understandable in light of her experiential background of developing, directing, and teaching within academic settings. In a 1973 publication, Daubenmire and King describe the undergraduate nursing curriculum at The Ohio State University which is based on King's original model as introduced in 1971. They contend that selection of a theoretical framework for curriculum development establishes boundaries of the systems to be studied, as well as the process involved (p 173, 1973). The 1981 refinement of King's model has explicated additional concepts as substantive content for nursing which could be meaningfully incorporated into educational programs.

Relationship to Nursing Practice

The relationship of King's model to practice is clear. Following the definition of each concept, King discusses either the concept's application to nursing or its implications for nursing. The primary focus of these discussions is professional practice. The theory of goal attainment derived from King's model describes human interactions manifested when nurses use the nursing process. Previously in this chapter, the significance of the model and the theory has been critiqued in terms of usefulness for clinical practice.

King presents the GONR as a means of documenting both process and outcomes when applying the theory of goal attainment in concrete nursing situations. The five major elements of the GONR are: 1) data base; 2) a problem list; 3) a goal list; 4) a plan; and, 5) progress notes (King, pp 164-165, 1981). Through systematic observations and measurements, the data base is collected. Disturbances, problems, or concerns of the patient make up the problem list. Short-term and long-term goals are mutually set by nurse and patient. The process/plans used to achieve these goals are documented in progress notes. Outcomes are identified as goals attained which constitute measures of effectiveness of care. King suggests that this approach "provides a built-in quality assurance system" (p 177, 1981).

When explaining how the GONR might be used within the nursing process, King presents an example of a patient with a medical diagnosis of cerebral vascular accident (pp 169-176, 1981). The following example demonstrates this writer's application of the theory and GONR format in a psychiatric/mental health setting. This example is presented as one illustration of the generalizability of King's formulations to another practice setting.

> Nurse and patient meet on an acute in-patient unit. Each perceives, acts, and reacts to the other in a reciprocally contingent manner. That is, the behavior of the nurse influences that of the patient and vice versa. The patient is perceived as being in need of assistance to restore and maintain mental health. The nurse is perceived as sincere, competent, and wanting to help. The major problem of anxiety is identified. Through interaction, mutually agreed upon goals are set and means to achieve the same are planned:

Problem: Anxiety

Goal 1. Explore causes of anxiety
Process: a. encourage expression of feelings
            b. allow patient to share at his/her own pace
            c. identify anxiety-producing situations
            d. provide reassurance and support
Goal 2. Identify characteristic response to anxiety
Process: a. observe and record verbal and nonverbal communication
            b. assess coping skills
Goal 3. Determine whether or not identified sources of anxiety can be avoided
Goal 4. Explore alternative means of reducing anxiety
Process: a. discourage repression of feelings
            b. help patient recognize and label anxiety
            c. educate how mild or moderate anxiety can be channeled positively/constructively
            d. teach verbal skills of assertion useful in counteracting anxiety responses

    e. practice role playing to reduce anxiety about new roles or situations

Progress of the purposeful interaction of nurse and patient is continually monitored. If the identified goals are attained, transaction will have occurred.

SUMMARY

In the words of Kaplan, "it seems impossible to formulate *all* the evidence and arguments that might be adduced to support or criticize a theory"; and, at any given moment, a particular theory will be accepted by some scientists and not by others (pp 311-312, 1964). Internal analysis and evaluation of King's model identified a few areas where logical adequacy was questioned. Any problems however, may be due, in part, to the broad scope and complexity of the framework. Nevertheless, the 1981 text demonstrates a substantial refinement of King's original (1971) formulations. The model has been evaluated as being very significant for nursing and having great potential to generate new information relevant to the discipline. Finally, external analysis has shown King's nursing model to have pragmatic value in relationship to research, education and practice.

REFERENCES

Anderson R, Carter I: Human Behavior in the Social Environment: A Systems Approach. Aldine Publishing Co., Chicago, Illinois, 1974

Code for nurses with interpretive statements. American Nurses' Association, Kansas City, Missouri, 1976

Daubenmire MJ, King IM: Nursing process model: A systems approach. Nursing Outlook, Vol 21, pp 512-517, 1973

Donaldson S, Crowley D: The discipline of nursing. Nursing Outlook, Vol 2, pp 113-120, 1978

Dubin R: Theory Building. The Free Press, New York, 1969

Ellis R: Characteristics of significant theories. Nursing Research, Vol 17, No 3, pp 217-222, 1968

Hardy M: Theories: Components, development, evaluation. Nursing Research, Vol 23, pp 100-107, 1974

Kaplan A: The Conduct of Inquiry. Chandler Publishing Co., San Francisco, California, 1964

King IM: Nursing theory: Problems and prospect. Nursing Science, pp 394-403, 1964

King IM: A conceptual frame of reference for nursing. Nursing Research, Vol 17, pp 27-30, 1968

King IM: Toward a Theory for Nursing. John Wiley & Sons, Inc., New York, 1971

King IM: The "why" of theory development. *In* Theory Development: What, Why, How? National League for Nursing, New York, 1978

King IM: A Theory for Nursing. John Wiley & Sons, Inc., New York, 1981

Reynolds PD: A Primer in Theory Construction. Bobbs-Merrill Co., Inc., New York, 1971

Satir V: Conjoint Family Therapy. Science & Behavior Books, Inc., Palo Alto, California, 1967

Standards for nursing practice. American Nurses' Association, Kansas City, Missouri, 1973

von Bertalanffy LL: General systems theory and psychiatry: An overview. *In* Gray W, Duhl F, Rizzo N (eds): General Systems Theory and Psychiatry, Little, Brown & Co., pp 33-50, 1969

Watzlawick P, Beavin J, Jackson D: Pragmatics of Human Communication. W.W. Norton & Company, Inc., New York, 1971

Weed L: Medical Records, Medical Education, and Patient Care. Case Western University Press, Cleveland, Ohio, 1969

14

MARTHA ROGERS' MODEL

Stephanie I. Muth Quillin & Judith Aumente Runk

INTRODUCTION

Martha Rogers began college in 1931 at the University of Tennessee, studying science for two years. She completed her nursing preparation at George Peabody College and received a master's degree from Teacher's College, Columbia University in 1945 in public health nursing. She held numerous leadership positions in public health nursing. In 1952 she earned the M.P.H. at Johns Hopkins University. In 1954 she earned her doctorate, an ScD, also from Johns Hopkins University. In the same year she went to New York University where she became Professor and Head of the Division of Nurse Education at New York University.

Rogers has received numerous awards, honors, and citations both nationally and internationally. Her colleagues consider her to be one of the most original thinkers in nursing. She continues to write and lecture extensively on nursing. Her contributions to the nursing literature are well known and extensively cited. The fact that Rogers values education, clear and creative thinking, and service to society and mankind is reflected in her writings. Her model of nursing, her abstract conceptual system, and her more specific theories for nursing have grown out of her effort to define, defend, and promote growth for nursing as a learned profession, one which is capable of responsible service to mankind. In her clear delineation of the scientific focus for nursing,

Rogers has had a most significant influence upon current scientific inquiry and professional nursing practice.

Rogers' model was first published in 1970 in her book, *An Introduction to the Theoretical Basis of Nursing*. Since then, major clarifications have been made as the conceptualizations have been further refined. These changes can be found in Rogers' chapter of *Conceptual Models for Nursing Practice* by Riehl and Roy (1980) and her series of six videotapes entitled *Nursing: The Science of Unitary Man* (Rogers, 1980b). The model has served as the basis for explication of other nursing conceptualizations, including those of Newman, Parse, and Fitzpatrick which are presented in subsequent chapters.

BASIC CONSIDERATIONS
INCLUDED IN THE MODEL

The basic considerations in any model are the building blocks or concepts. (These are also referred to as "units" by Dubin, 1978.) The basic considerations common to all the nursing models (nursing, persons, health and environment) will be defined first, then the concepts unique to Rogers' model will be described. Rogers uses the term "man" to refer to persons and humankind; thus when she is quoted directly, the term man is used.

Definitions of Nursing, Persons, Health, and Environment

Nursing

Rogers' (1970, 1980a) definition of nursing is a reflection of her humanistic concept of person and nursing. (Humanism is defined here as any system of thought or action which is concerned with the interests and ideals of people). The focus of nursing is compassionate concern for maintaining and promoting health, preventing illness and caring for and rehabilitating the sick and the disabled (Rogers, p vii, 1970). Rogers is committed to nursing as both a science with its abstract body of knowledge and an art which uses the science's body of knowledge. Professional practice in nursing "seeks to promote symphonic interaction between man and environment, to strengthen the coherence and integrity of the human field, and to direct and redirect patterning of the human and environmental fields for realization of maximum health potential" (Rogers, p 122, 1970).

Rogers states that the science of nursing is "the science of unitary man" (1980b). By this she means that no other science studies person as a whole. Nursing is the only science that deals with the whole person.

Person

Rogers' (1970, 1980b) view of person is characterized by a synthesis of knowledge from the physical, biological, and social sciences. Critical to her discussion is the statement that ". . . the whole cannot be understood when reduced to particulars" (p 44, 1970). Rogers states that the person's fundamental unit is not the cell but the human energy field. Person is understood within Rogers' conceptual model as a whole that is more than and different from the sum of its parts (Rogers, p 91, 1970). This holistic view of person has been part of nursing's history. Rogers has explicitly defined this concept in scientific terms. Person, defined by Rogers as an open system, is continually exchanging energy with the open system that is the environment. "Unitary man" is defined by Rogers (1980) as "a four-dimensional, negentropic energy field identified by pattern and organization and manifesting characteristics and behaviors that are different from those of the parts which cannot be predicted from knowledge of the parts" (p 332).

Rogers' primary concern is that nurses view the person not as a sum of parts but as a whole which is more than the sum of the parts. Persons are viewed optimistically, taking into account their capacity to change and their ability to participate creatively in change (1980b).

Environment

In Rogers' view each unique human field is extended to include its unique environmental field. "Unitary man" and environment are integral with each other and "coextensive with the universe." Rogers draws her concept of environment from von Bertalanffy and others who question the failure of physical laws to explain evolution of life. The term 'negentropy' comes from general systems theory to mean increasing order, complexity and heterogeneity (Rogers, 1970). The boundaries of environment become non-existent in Rogers' model since they extend to infinity. The person and the environment continuously exchange energy, resulting in mutual change. Rogers (1980) defines environment as "a four-dimensional, negentropic energy field identified by pattern and organization and encompassing all that (is) outside any given human field" (p 332). Rogers traces the history of human thought regarding the interaction of persons and environment (1970, 1980b). She concludes that the most logical conceptualization is that of a four-dimensional universe of interacting wholes.

Health

The word health is used often by Rogers but she declines to give it a specific definition. She has come to understand that illness and health are value words, broadly defined by each culture "to denote behaviors that are of high value and low value" (1980b). Rogers conceptualizes health and illness as expressions of the interaction of person and environment in the process of unfolding (pp 42, 51, 85, 1970).

Rogers considers health to be a value, defined by cultures and individuals. Her own use of the word in sentences is semantically compatible with definitions which connote wellness and absence of major illness or disease.

Description of Nursing Activity or Nursing Process

Rogers (1970) sees nursing activity as creative and imaginative, rooted in abstract knowledge, intellectual judgment, and compassion. She emphasizes the use of the nurse's own self combined with the safe utilization of the skills and technology of the time. Rogers' conceptual system specifies the unidirectional growth and development and rhythmical complexity of persons. Nursing process uses this system in assessing persons for a more flexible approach to health promotion. Nursing activity which includes nursing assessment, intervention, and rehabilitative services "is predicated upon the wholeness of man and derives its safety and effectiveness from a unified concept of human functioning. Nursing is concerned with evaluating the simultaneous states of the individual (or group) and the environment, and the preceding configurations leading up to the present" (Rogers, p 124, 1970).

Nursing process takes on a dynamism when viewed in the above framework. Instead of the static, time-limited goals set by the nurse for the person, Rogers proposes continuously evolving goal-setting that includes the nurse as an environmental component. Nursing is concerned with all people in all settings (Rogers, 1980b).

Interrelationships Among Concepts of Person, Environment, Health and Nursing

These four basic concepts are used in nursing models to explain or define nursing as a profession. Rogers sees nursing as a "learned profession" with full professional status (1980a, 1980b). This means that nursing not only has a practice component but that it is also a science.

Figure 14.1 illustrates an interpretation by the authors of the relationships between the four basic components as they are found in Rogers' publications. Also represented in the figure are the concepts that are unique to Rogers' model. As shown, concepts derived from study and observation about humankind provide a basis for the conceptual model. The conceptual model (discussed more completely later in this chapter) provides a stimulus for and gives direction to nursing science. The conceptual model also provides direction for practitioners by indicating general goals.

Prescriptive level theories are not contained in the conceptual model.

It is the nursing science that can, through research and theory development, provide explanatory, predictive, and prescriptive theories for nursing practice. Using a sound knowledge base derived from nursing science, nursing practice provides service to people which will maximize health potential. Service is seen by Rogers as rendered in all settings and appropriate for all people.

Description of the Other Basic Concepts that are Included

Rogers says that the basic "concepts or building blocks" of her conceptual model are: 1) energy fields; 2) openness; 3) pattern and organization; and, 4) four-dimensionality (1980a, 1980b).

Energy Fields

Rogers (1980a, 1980b) notes that current literature indicates that the fundamental unit of all living and non-living things is the energy field. Things do not *have* energy fields, rather they *are* energy fields. "Fundamental unit" connotes the representative

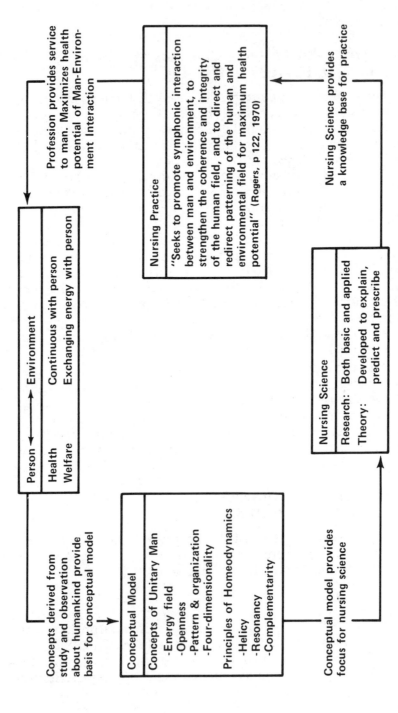

Figure 14.1. An Interpretation of Rogers' View of Nursing. Interrelationship among Man, Environment, Health, and Nursing.

unit of a thing which if examined thoroughly will reveal its character or nature. The cell was thought of as the fundamental unit of living things, but current research notes that the sum of all of the information about the functions and interactions of cells does not reveal the full nature of the organism. By labeling the energy field as the fundamental unit, Rogers hopes to avoid the "summing of parts" in nursing's study of man. Such "summing" results in views of man which are not helpful to nurses, such as mechanistic models, or models in which the mind and body are viewed separately. Rather Rogers hopes to promote a conceptualization of person which captures the essence of being in its entirely.

Openness

Rogers (1980a, 1980b) uses openness to refer to the qualities exhibited by an open system as opposed to a closed system. Open systems (energy fields) are conceptualized as extending to infinity and interacting with each other. Von Bertalanffy (1968) postulated that living systems are open systems which display negative entropy. In other words, living systems do not run down but instead display increasing diversity and complexity of organization. Rogers includes this view in her conceptual model.

Pattern And Organization

Since living things are always becoming more diverse, as well as interacting with their environments, the pattern of their wave organization is also constantly changing. Rogers (1970, 1980a, 1980b) views pattern and organization as characterizing the energy field that is the person and the environment. She views pattern and organization as unique and ever-changing.

Four-Dimensionality

This concept is the least clearly defined by Rogers. She states that words in our language are not sufficient to fully explain this concept. Rogers is using the concept of four-dimensionality proposed by Einstein and applying it in her model of person and environment. Neither Einstein nor Rogers view time as the fourth dimension. Rogers explains that the concept has to do with nonlinear time and non-static space which Einstein called spacetime (Roger, 1980b). Rogers prefers the term "four-dimensionality"

(1980a, 1980b). The relevance of this concept to the model is said by Rogers to be "a synthesis of non-linear coordinates from which innovative change continuously and evolutionally emerges" (1980a). Any present-point in this view is relative which has implications for the explanation of paranormal events (Rogers, 1980a).

Relationship of the Other Basic Concepts to Person, Environment, Health, and Nursing

The four concepts: energy fields, openness, pattern and organization, and four-dimensionality, when synthesized by Rogers, comprise "unitary man." Figure 14.1 illustrates that Rogers' four concepts are derived from study and observation of people (person-environment). They form the basis of nursing's abstract conceptual model which is ultimately related to nursing and health. The major components of the model of unitary man are discussed in the following sections.

Internal analysis and evaluation of the model will deal with analysis of Rogers' abstract conceptual system, rather than the model of nursing, health, and person displayed in Figure 14.1.

INTERNAL ANALYSIS OF THE MODEL

Underlying Assumptions

Rogers (1970) lists five assumptions underlying her conceptual model. They are derived from a selective review of the literature on man, physics, mathematics, and the behavioral sciences. They are:

1. Man is a unified whole possessing his own integrity and manifesting characteristics that are more than and different from the sum of his parts (p 47).
2. Man and environment are continuously exchanging matter and energy with one another (p 54).
3. The life process evolves irreversibly and unidirectionally along the space-time continuum (p 59).
4. Pattern and organization identify man and reflect his innovative wholeness (p 65).
5. Man is characterized by the capacity for abstraction and imagery, language and thought, sensation and emotion (p 73).

The first four assumptions have relevance for all living systems, as well as man. (Rogers, p 67, 1970) The fifth assumption applies only to man. The assumption differentiates man from the rest of the world of living things and places man at the height of evolutionary complexity of the living forms (p 67, 1970).

These assumptions are not restated in the 1980 publications, probably because they are subsumed elsewhere. The first assumption describing man as a unified whole which is more than the sum of parts is subsumed under the concept of energy fields. The second assumption, that of the mutual exchange of matter and energy, is discussed with the concept of openness. The third assumption which describes the life process evolving unidirectionally is actually a part of the principle of helicy. The fourth assumption regarding pattern and organization becomes the concept of pattern and organization. The fifth assumption, describing person as capable of abstract imagery, language, and thought, remains an adjunct to the current definition of person. It is clear that the concepts also function as assumptions.

Central Components of the Model

The central components of the model are unitary man and environment engaged in the life process. The components are derived from the synthesis of Rogers' four building blocks and comprise nursing's abstract conceptual system. The components are defined earlier in the chapter but are repeated here for clarity:

Unitary man: "a four-dimensional, negentropic energy field identified by pattern and organization and manifesting characteristics and behaviors that are different from those of the parts which cannot be predicted from knowledge of the parts" (Rogers, p 332, 1980a).

Environment: "a four-dimensional, negentropic energy field identified by pattern and organization and encompassing all that (is) outside any given human field" (p 332, 1980a).

From the abstract conceptual system, Rogers derives the three other components of the model. These are called principles of homeodynamics by Rogers; they are "broad generalizations that postulate the nature and direction of unitary human development" (p 333, 1980a).

The principle of helicy states:

The nature and direction of human and environmental change is continuously innovative, probabalistic and characterized by increasing diversity of human field and environmental field pattern and organization emerging out of the continuous mutual, simultaneous interaction between human and environmental field and manifesting non-repeating rhythmicities (Rogers, p 333, 1980a).

The principle of resonancy states:

The human field and the environmental field are identified by wave pattern and organization manifesting continuous change from lower frequency, longer wave patterns to higher frequency, shorter wave patterns (Rogers, p 333, 1980a).

The principle of complementarity states:

The interaction between human and environmental fields is continuous, mutual, simultaneous (Rogers, p 333, 1980).

Theories are also derived from the abstract conceptual system. They are the theories of: 1) accelerating evolution; 2) paranormal events; and, 3) rhythmical correlates of change (Rogers, 1980a).

Definitions of These Components

The components, man and environment, were defined earlier, as were helicy, resonancy, and complementarity. It should be noted that complementarity is subsumed into helicy but is stated separately by Rogers for purposes of clarity as well as to emphasize the non-causal nature of change. Rogers states that change is probabalistic. "Probabalistic" is an adjective, meaning "based on probabalism." Probabalism, in philosophy, is the doctrine that certainty in knowledge is impossible and that probability is a sufficient basis for action and belief.

The derived theories are defined below:

1. The theory of accelerating evolution: This theory states that change (evolution) is becoming more and more rapid. Rogers cites increasingly complex technology, changing sleep patterns, and changing blood pressure averages as examples (1980a).

2. Paranormal events: Rogers briefly explains that when human fields are viewed as four-dimensional (as well as

interacting) the relative present for one person is different from that of someone else. This could offer explanations for such phenomena as the well-documented instances of precognition as well as deja vu and clairvoyance (1980a).

3. Rhythmical correlates of change: This theory specifies that the wave patterns mentioned under resonancy include sleep/wake patterns, patterns of human field motion, and the developmental process of living and dying (1980a).

Relationships Among Components

Unitary man appears to be the most important component. Rogers emphasizes that man in his entirety is the focus of nursing's research and practice. Within the conceptual model man is defined as an energy field, inseparable from the environment and interchangable with his life process. In this sense man is the only component in the conceptual model; the principles serve to describe man. The derived theories are intended to explain, predict, and prescribe phenomena related to unitary man.

Analysis of Consistency

Dubin (1978) proposes a system for building or analyzing theories. He first relabels concepts as "units" which are things or variables "whose interactions constitute the subject matter of attention" (Dubin, p 7, 1978). He classifies and defines units. These definitions are useful in analyzing Rogers' abstract conceptual system.

According to Dubin's definitions, unitary man is a summative unit, standing for an entire complex thing. Summative units are very useful in "frames of reference" or "intellectual constructs" where they play a central role (p 79, 1978).

Helicy, resonancy, and complementarity may be conceptualized in Dubin's scheme as "laws of interaction" (p 89, 1978). As laws of interaction they describe the nature of change that is inevitable for the summative unit, unitary man. Helicy, resonancy, and complementarity state that change *emerges from* the man-environment interaction and is characterized by the *nature* of that interaction. "Emerges from" implies an ordering of events, namely that change follows interaction. This would allow helicy, resonancy, and complementarity to be defined as sequential laws.

Rogers refrains from use of words such as "follows" because they depend on a linear concept of time and connote a causal relationship. Dubin, however, states that sequence does *not* mean causation but merely our observation "that specified values of A are succeeded by specified values of B" (p 102, 1978). The linear concept of time is an inescapable reality for most researchers at this time, and thus sequential laws are useful without implying causation.

The efficiency of a law is its power to explain and predict about phenomena. "Where the range of unit values is broad, the law has low efficiency" (Dubin, p 109, 1978). The range of variability in Rogers' principles is broad, indicating a low range of efficiency. The beginning nature of theory development in nursing indicates that the level of efficiency of Rogers' principles is appropriate. The potential for more sophisticated development is inherent in the complexity of Rogers' conceptualizations.

Conceptual models are assessed in a variety of ways. Hardy (1978, 1974) and Ellis (1968) suggest examining scope, complexity, and usefulness. Rogers' model is broad in scope and centered on the life process of man. The theory is complex and treats multiple variables. The model suggests global hypotheses which may then be further modified and specified. The usefulness of the model to practice lies in its ability to relate multiple variables to the life process of man. Devising methods to measure the life process of man remains a challenge to researchers using the model. The model's linguistic complexity may lead to misinterpretation. Clear understanding of the model is necessary for those attempting to make the leap from the model to practice and education.

Testing of hypotheses derived from the model has been undertaken by several researchers in nursing. As this body of research continues to grow, examination of hypotheses and results will allow support, rejection, and/or modification of the model. Issues identified in use of the model are the complexity of its language, the need for those using the model to develop a noncausal mind-set, and the encompassing nature of its concepts, which allows for an unlimited inclusion of variables to be considered.

Analysis of Adequacy

According to Dubin (1978), "The argument about the adequacy of the theoretical model is always and only an argument about the logic employed in constructing it" (p 12, 1978). Using this standard, no flaws in logic can be found in the model. The model is logically consistent. Specific relationships between the three derived theories that Rogers mentions in the 1980 publications, (i.e., the theory of accelerating change, the theory of paranormal events, and the theory of rhythmical correlates of change) and the basic conceptualization of Rogers are currently being explicated. These theories must be further developed, however, before they can properly be examined and analyzed. It will be interesting to note further contributions to the continued refinement of Rogers' overall conceptualizations regarding unitary man.

EXTERNAL ANALYSIS OF THE MODEL

Relationship to Nursing Research

As shown in Figure 14.1, Rogers' conceptual model is directly related to research and theory development in nursing science. The conceptual model provides the stimulus and direction for these scientific activities. Rogers' model offers a way of looking at reality that is unique to the nursing profession. Researchers whose assumptions and propositions are consistent with the model are able to clearly defend their work as nursing. Rogers' delineation of the science of nursing provides a unique and substantive focus for the discipline.

Rogers (1967) indicates that the critical need in nursing is for basic research in the science of nursing. Rogers expects the theory emerging from her model to ultimately explain, predict, and prescribe about unitary man and life process phenomena (1980a). Hence there is a need for both basic and applied research (Rogers, 1980a). The model itself is not testable in itself nor is it meant to be. Rather, theories and hypotheses derived from the model are subjected to empirical test.

The derivation of testable theories or hypotheses from the model require understanding and inferences. Some researchers use the model as a beginning point for the generation of research; they may not relate their final product to the model because the relationship between the model and the research is general. However, as editors of nursing journals and nurses are becoming interested in the nursing models, more researchers and theorists are explicitly stating the connections between their work and Rogers' model. Examples of research related to Rogers' conceptualization include that of Newman (1978), Fawcett (1975), and Fitzpatrick (1980), as well as several presenters at the ANA Council of Nurse Researchers symposium entitled "Research related to Rogers'

Conceptual Model" (ANA Council of Nurse Researchers, Washington, D.C., September 16-18, 1981). Theorists who have extended Rogers' model to make it less vague, especially in the definition and understanding of health, are Fitzpatrick (1983), Newman (1979) and Parse (1981). These models are analyzed in subsequent chapters.

Relationship to Nursing Education

In 1963, Rogers called for the rebuilding of graduate and undergraduate programs in nursing to reflect the evolution of nursing science. In 1964 she outlined a doctoral program in nursing consistent with the science of unitary man. The conceptual framework is used as a guide for studying and learning. For example, students would take courses in physics and philosophy as well as the other more usual electives. She sees nursing more closely related to the liberal arts college than to any of the other colleges of the university. Education in Rogers' framework prepares a generalist in nursing who views man and environment as interacting and ever-changing.

A strength of Rogers' model in education is the conceptualization of nursing as a theory-based science. This conceptualization mandated university-based education for nurses and paved the way for the development of the doctor of philosophy degree in nursing, which is now a reality in many universities.

Another strength of Rogers' model is its arguments in favor of probability and against causality. This argument places theorists using the model in congruence with the most current concepts in scientific thought. Kerlinger (1973) and Dubin (1978) provide examples of this thinking. The practitioner of nursing may dislike the probability argument because it means giving up the fantasy that we can ever be absolutely certain that an intervention will be effective 100 percent of the time. The researcher in nursing may more readily accept the probability argument, recognizing that statistical methods reveal probabilities rather than certainties.

Relationship to Nursing Practice

Although Rogers sees the theory which derives from her conceptual model as translatable to practice, the examples she gives are general. She has not provided a specific framework for use in the nursing process. Falco and Lobo (1980) use helicy, resonancy, and complementarity to derive a care plan (assessment, diagnosis, implementation, evaluation) for a specific individual. The attempt is thoughtful and imaginative. The result of this application remains general rather than specific.

As depicted in Figure 14.1, Rogers' conceptual model can be used in research and theory development. It is the responsibility of the researcher and theorist to develop the specific knowledge base for practice. A general guideline for practitioners is interpreted by Newman:

> In calling for a new way of viewing man, as well as health and illness, Rogers' model does not require that one discard previous knowledge, but it does require that such knowledge be viewed differently. Disease conditions can no longer be considered as entities unto themselves but must be regarded as manifestations of the total pattern of the individual in interaction with the environment (p 21, 1979).

Rogers (1980a, 1980b) envisions changes in nursing practice based on the theories evolving from her model. For example, the aging process can be perceived not as a running down of the individual but as a growing diversity in field pattern and organization, such that many of the characteristics of older persons, as in changing sleep patterns, would cease to be viewed as abnormal or in need of intervention. Other changes she envisions are that dying be viewed as a process rather than an event; that nurses increase and formalize their use of touch; and that nursing care become even more individualized to specific persons in their own unique situations, rather than using mass criteria for large "clumps" of individuals.

SUMMARY

Rogers' abstract conceptual model is broad in scope. It treats the complexity of the single variable, the summative unit "unitary man." The model is not meant to be testable, but theories drawn from it are testable. While the abstract conceptual model may not be directly useful to practice it provides a substantive base for research and theory development which provides the knowledge base for practice. For Rogers, professional practice flows from the application of knowledge. The model generates information by increasing our understanding of man and the life process and by encouraging theory development and the delineation of testable hypotheses. Terminology is clear, although the new words (neologisms) sometimes seem difficult. These neologisms avoid confusion with terms from other fields. The sophisticated concepts and linkages require study and understanding.

Rogers' model is an optimistic and evolving one. Implicit and explicit values in Rogers' view of nursing are a high respect for individuals, and respect for values and characteristics of individuals and groups which may be "deviant" in the sense of "not with the average (norm)." Rogers' model challenges the researcher, the educator, and the practitioner to meet their societal obligations in creative ways. Martha Rogers has been instrumental in moving nursing towards full professionalization. Her conceptual model of unitary man presents a clear, direct statement about the unique focus of nursing, and a visionary perspective of nursing as science and art.

REFERENCES

Dubin R: Theory Building, The Free Press, New York, 1978

Duffey M, Muhlenkamp AF: A framework for theory analysis. Nursing Outlook, Vol 22, pp 570-547, 1974

Ellis R: Characteristics of significant theories. Nursing Research, Vol 17, No 3, pp 217-222, 1968

Falco SM, Lobo ML: Martha E. Rogers. In the Nursing Theories Conference Group, George JB (ed): Nursing theories: The base for professional nursing practice. Prentice-Hall, Inc., Englewood Cliffs, New Jersey, 1980

Fawcett J: The family as a living open system: An emerging conceptual framework for nursing. International Nursing Review, Vol 22, No 4, pp 113-116, 1975

Fitzpatrick JJ: Patients' perceptions of time: Current research. International Nursing Review, Vol 27, No 5, pp 148-153, 1980

Fitzpatrick JJ: A life perspective rhythm model. In Fitzpatrick JJ, Whall AL (eds): Conceptual Models of Nursing: Analysis and Application. Robert J. Brady Co., Bowie, Maryland, 1983

Greenwood E: Attributes of a profession. Social Work. Vol 2, No 3, pp 45-55, 1975

Hardy ME: Theories: components, development, evaluation. Nursing Research, Vol 23, pp 100-107, 1974

Hardy ME: Perspectives on nursing theory. Advances in Nursing Science, Vol 1, pp 37-48, 1978

Kaplan A: The Conduct of Inquiry. Chandler, Scranton, Pennsylvania, 1964

Kerlinger FN: Foundations of Behavioral Research (2nd ed). Holt, Rinehart & Winston, New York, 1973

Kuhn TS: The Structure of Scientific Revolutions. University of Chicago, Chicago, Illinois, 1962

Newman MA: Application of theory in education and service. Paper presented at the Nurse Educator Conference at New York University, New York, 1978

Newman MA: Theory Development in Nursing. F.A. Davis, Philadelphia, Pennsylvania, 1979

Parse RR: Man-living-health, a theory of nursing. John Wiley & Sons, Inc., New York, 1981

Popper KR: Conjectures and Refutations, the Growth of Scientific Knowledge. Basic Books, New York, 1962

Rogers ME: Building a strong educational foundation. American Journal of Nursing, Vol 63, No 6, pp 94-95, 1963

Rogers ME: Reveille in Nursing. F.A. Davis, Philadelphia, Pennsylvania, 1964

Rogers ME: Nursing science: Research and researchers. Paper presented at Annual Conference on Research and Nursing, Division of Nursing Education, Teachers College, Columbia University, New York, February 3, 1967

Rogers ME: The Theoretical Basis of Nursing. F.A. Davis, Philadelphia, Pennsylvania, 1970

Rogers ME: Nursing: A science of unitary man. In Riehl JP, Roy C (eds): Conceptual Models for Nursing Practice, 2nd ed. Appleton-Century-Crofts, New York, 1980a

Rogers ME: The science of unitary man. Media for Nursing (Videotape), New York, 1980b

von Bertalanffy L: General System Theory. George Braziller, Inc., New York, 1968

15

NEWMAN'S MODEL OF HEALTH

Veronica Engle

INTRODUCTION

Margaret Newman's interest in health, movement, and time originated in rehabilitation nursing practice. She noticed that individual's confined to bed described time as dragging (Newman, 1979). This observation was confirmed by studies that indicated degree of physical mobility as well as state of health influenced the perception of time.

She studied this relationship between movement and time at New York University using Martha Rogers' (1970) model for nursing. Her doctoral dissertation (Newman, 1971) examined the effect of changes in cadence (movement) on the perception of time, and laid the groundwork for future study (Newman, 1972, 1976). As a result of this research and the influence of Rogers' model for nursing, Newman refined and expanded her original conceptualization into her model of health.

BASIC CONSIDERATION

Nursing science is currently at an early stage of development. This is reflected in the various nursing models that view person, health, and environment in different ways. While these diverse viewpoints indicate that there is no one accepted view of nursing, nursing science must begin to define its focus (Donaldson and Crowley, 1978).

One approach to establishing the focus of nursing science is the development of criteria that theory must meet in order to have direct application to nursing. Newman (1979) suggests three criteria. Nursing theories should focus on the life process, aspects of the life process related to health, and actions facilitating health. Of these three criteria, Newman places the most emphasis on the action component when stating that nursing science is the "process of finding out how to facilitate the health of man" (Newman, p 7, 1979).

The focus of Newman's (1979) model is health. Therefore, less emphasis is placed on the other commonly accepted elements of nursing models (person, environment, nursing). Newman describes *person* and *environment* as part of the life process. The life process, however, is not clearly identified. The reader can assume that Newman's use of the life process is consistent with Rogers' (1970) model for nursing, because both Newman and Rogers emphasize the qualities of wholeness, pattern and organization, rhythmicity, and unidirectionality. Within the context of the life process, person and environment are defined as coextensive energy fields. Both person and environment evolve together, moving toward increasing complexity and diversity that is manifested by rhythmic patterns along the dimensions of space and time (Rogers, 1970).

Newman's (1979) description of nursing reflects the early stage of development of her model. She defines nursing as including nursing theory, nursing science, nursing action, and nursing goal. However, the dominant theme of nursing as health promotion is consistently used by Newman in her model of health. Newman (p 53, 1979) states that nursing theory "must specify and test actions necessary in order to promote health, the stated purpose of nursing." She also states that "the goal of nursing is not to make people well, or to prevent their getting sick, but to assist people to utilize the power that is within them as they evolve toward higher levels of consciousness" (Newman, p 67, 1979).

The definition and discussion of *health* by Newman (1979) is the most complex, as well as the most fully developed. This approach is consistent with Newman's stated purpose of defining the focus of nursing via "a precise conceptualization of the nature of health ... in order to specify theory which relates to that phenomenon" (Newman, p 55, 1979). Health is defined in four ways. First, health is a fusion of disease and non-disease. There is a condition specified as disease, whereas its opposite is called non-disease. "The fusion of the two antithetical concepts brings forth a synthesis, which can be regarded as health" (Newman, p 56, 1979). The fusion eliminates the current dichotomy between health and illness, and produces a holistic definition of health.

Second, health is defined as an individual's unique pattern. This pattern is basic to the person, and exists prior to structural or functional changes that may be manifested as pathology. If illness is the only way for an individual's pattern to manifest itself, then illness becomes health for that individual. Health, therefore, encompasses both illness and pathology, and reflects the synthesis of disease and non-disease.

In addition to the two previous definitions, health is further defined as both the expansion of consciousness as well as the totality of the life process. This relationship of health to expanded consciousness and to the life process is unclear because both health and life process are summative units. A summative unit has "the property that derives from the interaction of a number of other properties" (Dubin, p 67, 1978). As a result, the exact nature of the relationship of health to its four definitions (disease—non-disease, basic pattern, expanded consciousness, life process) cannot be precisely determined because the definitions of health are interrelated, rather than discrete.

Rather than focus on health per se, Newman (1979) elaborates on a limited number of phenomena of the life process. Four concepts, *movement, time, space,* and *consciousness,* provide a framework from which to view health (see Figure 15.1). These concepts, as the previous four definitions of health, are interrelated and summative units:

1. Time and space have a complementary relationship.
2. Movement is a means whereby space and time become a reality.
3. Movement is a reflection of consciousness.
4. Time is a function of movement.
5. Time is a measure of consciousness (Newman, p 60, 1979).

Of these four concepts, Newman places the greatest emphasis on consciousness, and describes health as expanded consciousness.

The figure that Newman (1979) uses to illustrate the interrelationships among the four concepts does not clearly illustrate the complexity of her definition of health (see Figure 15.1). It could be revised to include three, three-dimensional concentric

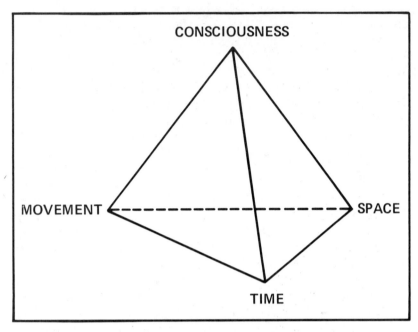

Figure 15.1. Interrelationships of Phenomena of the Life Process. (*From:* Newman M: Theory Development. F.A. Davis Co., Philadelphia, Pennsylvania, p 60, 1979. With permission of F.A. Davis Co.)

figures (see Figure 15.2). The small sphere in the center of the pyramid represents health, the focus of inquiry. A line connects the small sphere to the consciousness vertex of the pyramid. The other vertexes of the pyramid represent the relationship of movement, time, space, and consciousness to each other. This pyramid, in turn, is encompassed by a larger sphere representing the totality of the life process. Thus, the interrelationships among the four definitions of health are clarified.

When analyzing each of the four concepts separately, note that movement, time, space, and consciousness are summative units used to provide a general focus to orient the reader, rather than to provide specific definitions (Dubin, 1978). Accordingly, the definitions of the four concepts reflect this general focus. These concepts provide insight into a new way of viewing health, and reflect the influence of Rogers' (1970) model for nursing.

The first concept, *movement,* is defined as "an essential property of matter," incorporating both "awareness of self (and) a means of communication" (Newman, p 62, 1979). Movement is further described as occurring between the two states of rest in the action-rest cycle. Movement patterns may take place at the microscopic level, such as nerve action potentials, or at the macroscopic level, such as everyday activities. Each individual has a unique pattern of movement that is a holistic measure of the interaction between the person and environment.

The second concept, *time*, is defined only as the experience of time. Newman (1979) does not elaborate beyond that definition to include other parameters of temporal experience, such as duration. The third concept, *space*, is defined in multiple ways: three-dimensional space, life space, personal space, and inner space.

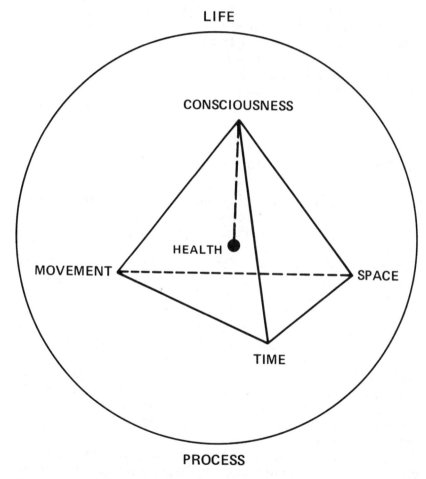

Figure 15.2. Engle's Representation of Newman's Model of Health.

Further discussion of the two concepts, time and space, is in terms of their complementary relationship, because "the concept of space . . . is inextricably linked to the concept of time" (Newman, p 61, 1979). The world is viewed in terms of dynamic patterns of activity having both space and time, as well as movement aspects. Space-time patterns are macroscopic, such as black holes, or microscopic, such as everyday events.

The fourth and last concept, *consciousness*, like the three preceding concepts, is defined in terms of more than one parameter. Consciousness refers to the left and right hemispheres of the brain, as well as to age and time. Dimensions of consciousness are illustrated by the left hemisphere's "analytical, sequence-perceiving processes (and the right hemisphere's) synthesis-oriented, symbolic intuitive modes" (Newman, p 65, 1979). Consciousness may also be defined in terms of the relationship of age to time, measured by the Consciousness Index. The Consciousness Index is defined by Newman (1979) as the ratio of the individual's perception of clock time (subjective time) to actual clock time (objective). This Index has been found to increase with age (Newman, 1979).

INTERNAL ANALYSIS

The internal analysis of Newman's (1979) model addresses six areas: 1) assumptions; 2) central components and importance; 3) relationships among concepts; 4) specificity; 5) adequacy; and 6) significance. The *assumptions* of Newman's model for health, derived from Rogers' (1970) model for nursing, refer to person, environment, and their interaction with each other. Person and environment are open systems as well as energy fields. In particular, the person is capable of abstraction, thought, sensation, and emotion. The characteristics of person are greater than the sum of his/her parts. Both person and environment are continuously, mutually, and simultaneously interacting with each other. Characteristics of this interaction include pattern and organization, rhythmicity, unidirectionality, and increasing diversity and complexity. These characteristics are most evident in Newman's descriptions and definitions of health, movement, time, space, and consciousness.

The concepts of movement, time, space, and consciousness are the *central components* of the model. All four concepts are summative units, described in relationship to health as well as to each other. At first reading, all four concepts appear equally *important*. This equality is demonstrated by the pyramid (see Figure 15.1) in which all concepts are weighted equally in order to provide a unified approach to health. Upon reanalysis of Newman's (1979) four definitions of health, consciousness becomes the most important concept because health is defined as expanded consciousness. This weighting of consciousness is illustrated in Figure 15.2, in which consciousness assumes a central role in defining health while still related to movement, time, and space.

The *relationships* among the concepts are described by symmetrical, categorical laws in which "values of one unit are associated with values of another unit" (Dubin, p 98, 1978). These relationships, or linkages among the concepts, can never rise above the lowest level of efficiency in predicting as well as understanding health. Although the linkages lack efficiency, Newman's (1979) model of health may be considered powerful because it distinguishes a limited number of concepts (four) and focuses on one realm, health (Dubin, 1978).

Newman's (1979) model may be classified as a grand theory, although it is less abstract than Rogers' (1970) model for nursing. The characteristics of a grand theory are in accord with the stated purpose of Newman's model, to provide a focus for theory development. The model, therefore, is not at a level of *specificity* that would be considered a theoretical structure. It provides a general orientation that is characteristic of a conceptualization at its early stage of development (Hardy, 1978).

A fifth area for internal analysis is *adequacy*, logical as well as empirical (Hardy, 1974). Newman's (1979) model has limited logical adequacy because the central components (movement, time, space, consciousness) are summative units. The model likewise has little empirical adequacy, because the central components are not defined operationally. This, however, is consistent with the aim of the model, which is to identify an area for development of integrated theories from which testable hypotheses can be derived.

The final aspect of internal analysis is *significance*, or the scope and complexity of a model or theory. Ellis (1968) states that a theory has scope if the concepts are linked in a framework with a broad area of concern. Newman's (1979) model, therefore, is broad in scope because it contains four central components that all relate to health. Complexity refers to the number of variables and relationships. The model is likewise complex because all of the central components are interrelated. Thus this model, health, has a high level of significance.

EXTERNAL ANALYSIS

External analysis addresses the impact of the model on research, education, and practice. The role of *research* is twofold: to test theory as well as to establish a scientific knowledge base from which to practice professional nursing. The relationship between research and theory in nursing science has not always been present in the past. Consequently, there is limited integration of theories, studies are not related to each other, and knowledge is fragmented. One exception, however, is the numerous studies of movement and time by nurse researchers.

Nurse researchers have studied movement in a variety of ways, such as motor abilities (Barnard, 1973); tempo (Newman, 1976; Tompkins, 1980); gross motor limb activity (Chapman, 1978; Downs and Fitzpatrick, 1976); and movement therapy (Goldberg and Fitzpatrick, 1980). Time has been studied primarily as time perception (Engle, 1981; Smith, 1979) and temporal perspective (Fitzpatrick and Donovan, 1978). The conceptual model for these studies was either Rogers' (1970) model for nursing or Newman's (1979) model for health.

The beauty of using Newman's (1979) model as the conceptual framework for research lies in its general focus on health, from which multiple propositions can be derived. The focus, based on the concepts of movement, time, space, and consciousness, is not limited by current nursing practice (Phillips, 1977) and provides a new way of viewing health via these nontraditional concepts. Newman's model, therefore, provides a future, rather than a present orientation toward the study of health.

Propositions from Newman's (1979) model of health have been studied intensively. That is, attention has focused on a limited number of strategic propositions (Dubin, 1978). Research investigated the relationship between movement and time in predominantly college-aged men and women (Newman, 1971, 1972, 1976; Tompkins, 1980), as well as in older women (Engle, 1981). In all five studies, movement tempo was negatively related to time perception. In addition, the postulated influence of age on the Consciousness Index was supported in the studies of women.

These studies using Newman's (1979) model for health illustrate the value of intensive testing of propositions. Use of the same model of health and similar methodologies permitted comparison of findings across studies in order to demonstrate the effect of age on movement tempo and time perception. Consequently, a cohesive body of knowledge is being developed on the relationship between movement and time across different age groups.

Extensive tests of a greater number of propositions (Dubin, 1978) derived from Newman's (1979) model of health have not been done. This may be due to the recent publication of Newman's model of health, or the nature of the model itself. The summative units (movement, time, space, consciousness) have a limited number of empirical indicators. It is therefore difficult to test all of the relationships among concepts at this time. In addition, traditional methodologies may not be sufficient to examine the propositions, because the model is future-oriented and visionary. The focus of study may need to shift from many cases at one time, to few cases over an extended period of time. This method is necessary in order to delineate patterns over time. The type of research may, likewise, need to shift to descriptive, intuitive, historical, or philosophical studies.

Just as research tests theory, it also establishes a scientific knowledge base for nursing education and nursing practice. Roy (p 17, 1979) states that "the function of nursing *education* (is) the development and sharing of knowledge concerning the theories about the phenomena of nursing and the knowledge and skills related to the theories of the practice of nursing." Currently, few curricula are based on nursing models, with no curriculum (as far as can be determined) based on Newman's (1979) model of health. Health, however, is a traditional component in nursing curricula and Newman's model could provide an alternative view of health. Therefore, the potential use of Newman's model in education is great, due to its many-faceted conceptualization of health.

Nursing *practice* utilizes the scientific knowledge base unique to nursing science, as well as knowledge derived from other disciplines. The knowledge base derived from Newman's (1979) conceptualization of health is potentially useful because it builds on concepts, movement and time, already familiar to nurses. Movement and time are historically an intrinsic part of nursing interventions, although not explicitly identified. For example, bed rest and its concomitant complications result from decreased movement of body fluids (sputum, urine, blood, feces) or body structures (joints, muscles). Nursing interventions based on movement, such as range of motion exercises, ambulation, and deep breathing and coughing, prevent or alleviate these alterations. Likewise, time is an important parameter because nurse-client interactions, self health-care activities, or nursing interventions take place throughout a 24-hour period of time.

Research findings indicate that movement tempo as measured by cadence, and time perception as measured by perceived duration, may be particularly relevant for gerontological nursing practice (Engle, 1981). Cadence is an easy to use, unobtrusive, inexpensive measure of health. It could be used in selected clinical experiences, such as before or after surgery. Measurement of cadence before surgery would provide a baseline from which to compare post-operative cadence and return to health. Perception of time is the second area for nursing assessment because time passes faster for older people. Nurses may need to use a slower pace when communicating or providing physical care, allowing more time for the (seemingly slower) older client to respond.

SUMMARY

In summary, Newman's (1979) model provides a unique focus on health, from which testable theories can be derived. The concepts used to describe health (movement, time, space, consciousness) are visionary, and reflect a model that is both broad in scope and complex, yet of limited logical and empirical adequacy. A small number of studies using Newman's model have been done, although the model provides fertile ground for the future development of a knowledge base unique to nursing science.

REFERENCES

Barnard R: Field-dependence/independence and selected motor abilities. Unpublished doctoral dissertation, New York University, New York, 1973

Chapman J: The relationship between auditory stimulation and gross motor activity of short-gestation infants. Research in Nursing and Health, Vol 1, pp 29-36, 1978

Donaldson S, Crowley D: The discipline of nursing. Nursing Outlook, Vol 2, pp 113-120, 1978

Downs F, Fitzpatrick J: Preliminary investigation of the reliability and validity of a tool for the assessment of body position and motor activity. Nursing Research, Vol 25, pp 404-408, 1976

Dubin R: Theory Building. The Free Press, New York, 1978

Ellis R: Characteristics of significant theories. Nursing Research, Vol 17, No 3, pp 217-222, 1968

Engle V: A study of the relationship between self-assessment of health, function, personal tempo and time perception in elderly women. Unpublished doctoral dissertation, Wayne State University, Detroit, Michigan, 1981

Fitzpatrick J, Donovan M: Temporal experience and motor behavior among the aging. Research in Nursing and Health, Vol 1, pp 60-68, 1978

Goldberg W, Fitzpatrick J: Movement therapy and the aged. Nursing Research, Vol 29, pp 339-346, 1980

Hardy M: Theories: Components, development, evaluation. Nursing Research, Vol 23, pp 100-107, 1974

Hardy M: Evaluating nursing theory. In Theory Development: What, Why, How? National League for Nursing, pp 75-86, New York, 1978

Newman M: An investigation of the relationship between gait tempo and time perception. Unpublished doctoral dissertation, New York University, New York, 1971

Newman M: Time estimation in relation to gait tempo. Perceptual and Motor Skills, Vol 34, pp 359-366, 1972

Newman M: Movement tempo and the experience of time. Nursing Research, Vol 25, pp 273-279, 1976

Newman M: Theory Development in Nursing. F.A. Davis Co., Philadelphia, Pennsylvania, 1979

Phillips J: Nursing systems and nursing models. Image, Vol 9, pp 4-7, 1977

Rogers M: An introduction to the theoretical basis of nursing. F.A. Davis Co., Philadelphia, Pennsylvania, 1970

Roy C: Relating nursing theory to education: A new era. Nurse Educator, pp 16-21, March-April, 1979

Smith M: Duration experience for bed-confined subjects: A replication and refinement. Nursing Research, Vol 28, pp 139-144, 1979

Tompkins E: Effect of restricted mobility and dominance in perceived duration. Nursing Research, Vol 29, pp 333-338, 1980

16

PARSE'S THEORY OF NURSING

S. Joy Winkler

INTRODUCTION

Parse's expressed intent in developing her theory of Man-Living-Health is to contribute to the unique body of knowledge underlying practice. It represents a significant example of the influence of Rogers' (1970) nursing model upon later nurse theorists. Parse's theory is deductively derived from Rogers and the existential-phenomenological philosophers Heidegger, Sartre, and Merleau-Ponty. Parse's definition of a theory of nursing reflects these sources: "a system of interrelated concepts describing the unitary man's interrelating with the environment while cocreating health" (p 13). While Dubin (1978) states that the term theory may be used interchangeably with model, others observe that a model becomes a theory only when validated. Therefore, it seems more appropriate at this stage of its development to call Parse's theory a model.

BASIC CONSIDERATIONS

Theories and models are built from concepts. Because of the many associated meanings for this term, in analysis of a theory it is essential to focus on the meaning given each concept by its relation to other concepts (Hardy, 1974). Given the existentialist-phenomenonological underlying premise of "all at once" (Barrett,

1964), the delineation of the separate definitions of person, environment, health, and nursing from Parse's contruct of Man-Living-Health is somewhat difficult. While each major concept is defined in terms of the others, the definitions are not circular. The process of interrelating conveys a complexity and multiplicity of meanings consistent with the philosophical origins of the model. In reading Parse, it is helpful to keep in mind that phenomenology is concerned with temporality, existentialism with freedom (Bannan, 1967).

Nursing

Parse views nursing as a science and an art, rooted in the human rather than the natural sciences. She does not give as clear an explication of this basic concept as she does of person, environment and health. Nursing's focus is "man as living unity . . . man's qualitative participation with health experiences" (Parse, p 4, 1981a). The responsibility of nursing in its practice is "guiding the choosing of possibilities in the changing health process . . . through intersubjective participation with persons and their families" (Parse, p 81, 1981a). These statements are consistent with and a refining of her definition of nursing in an earlier work: "Nursing is a human science profession concerned with the care of unitary man as he evolves from conception to death" (Parse, p 7, 1974). Foci of nursing practice include: the illumination of the "unique ways . . . generational and contemporary family . . . patterns of interrelating . . . cocreate lived values . . . in reflectively choosing viewpoints relative to the possibilities available in the changing health process" and "changing priorities in lived value" (Parse, p 81, 82, 1981a). This process involves the concurrent mobilization of individual and family energies for cocreation. It should be noted that family refers to those with whom one is closely connected. Nursing as a social service directed towards persons collectively is not specifically addressed. Such an omission is consistent with the existential emphasis on the individual (Barrett, 1964). The apparent rejection of the need for natural science knowledge to the understanding and care of unitary man seems to negate the biophysical phenomena integral to the holistic view of person.

Parse's definition of nursing practice is reflective of the existentialist-phenomenological view of man being and becoming in the process of relating (Barrett, 1964). It is also reflective of Rogers' (1980) view of the interaction of person and environment. Parse's explicit acknowledgement that persons' values learned in their familial and cultural milieus affect health and, therefore, nursing practice is a strength of her concept of nursing. Also of significance is the specification of the nurse's role in guiding persons to assume responsibility for health, an increasingly strong theme in current health and nursing literature. Absence of specific reference to the nurse's role in the prevention of illness and restoration of health may be unacceptable to some nurses. Her philosophical perspective is particularly evident in the language and style of her final statement on nursing. The unfamiliarity of usage of words may prove puzzling to some:

> Nursing is unfolding in simultaneous mutual interchange with the world transcending with greater diversity and complexity ... is all at once what it was, is, and will become, growing evermore explicit but always with the mystery of the not yet (Parse, p 172, 1981a).

As will be seen, this is a parallel description to that given for person.

Person

The centrality of the concept of person to Parse's model is evident in this it is implicit or explicit in all concepts, assumptions, and principles. Ellis (1968) notes that the person (patient) is the essential unit in the interrelationship of units in theories significant for nursing. The fundamental tenet or principle underlying Parse's definition of person is that she/he participates in her/his health. "... Unitary man ... coparticipates with the environment in creating and becoming, is whole, open and free to choose ways of living health" (Parse, p 7, 1981a). This broad definition is derived from the existential-phenomenological tenents or principles of intentionality and human subjectivity, and the concepts of coconstitution, coexistence, and situated freedom. Rogers' (1980) principles of helicy, resonancy, and complementarity, and concepts of energy field, openness, pattern and organization, and four dimensionality, also form the basis of Parse's deduction of this concept. They are the basis as well of the concepts of health and environment. The philosophical understanding of the person will be elaborated first.

Intentionality is the giving of particular meaning and significance (Bannan, 1967). The person's becoming over time reflects connections with predecessors and contemporaries (historicity), the givens to which one is born and one's immediate situation (facticity). Situated freedom, the concept stating that the person both chooses her/his attitude to life situations, and plays a part in choosing these situations, emerges from this tenet. One is responsible both for one's choices and their consequences, even those unknown at the time of decision. The other concept arising from this tenet is that of coexistence, the person as an emerging being in the world with others. In choosing among the possibles which become actuals, a person lives values, transcends the present to reach beyond self, and cocreates the world. Human subjectivity refers to the person as "a unity of the subject world relationship" (Parse, p 19, 1981a). The person's relationship with the world is such that the two parts together create a whole greater than and different from the person and her/his world seen separately. The person interrelates with others and their various world views, thus creating the meaning of any situation. Because the person is aware of the possibility of non-being, loss of self in dying, she/he is aware of losing affirmation of life through choices.

The relationship of Rogers' principles and concepts to Parse's concept of person may be explained as follows: "(the person) is rhythmically becoming through continuous open energy interchange with the environment . . . unitary process of negentropically unfolding as (the person) chooses health possibilities (Parse, pp 30, 39, 1981a) . . . in pattern and organization is distinct from the pattern and organization of the environment" (Parse, p 26, 1981a). In the continuous interchange of energy with others and the environment, transcendence occurs, and the person in aging moves toward greater complexity and diversity. The person's experiencing is affected by relative time-space boundaries or interfaces where energy interchanges occur, and as space time energy events do not repeat themselves "man as relative present is more than and different from before" (Parse, p 33, 1981a).

Environment

Parse treats person-environment as a construct, making it difficult to explicate the concept of environment separately. This is consistent with Rogers' (1970) exposition of person-environment as inseparable, complementary, evolving together, coextensive with each other and the universe. It is also in harmony with the existentialist view of person being in the world all at once and together (Barrett, 1964). From the phenomenological context, everything that shows itself to the person in whatever form it may be, constitutes the environment (Kockelmans, 1965). Hence, the internal and external environments are not delineated separately but together constitute everything coming into the person's awareness. Thus, the person is seen as "coparticipating with the environment in simultaneously evolving the individual patterns of relating that distinguish an individual from an environmental pattern..." (Parse, p 26, 1981a). The environment and the person rhythmically emerge together in the direction of greater complexity. The energy interchange of the environment with the person is relative and simultaneous at many levels, with an infinite number of universes existing simultaneously within each person's environment. The person with environment reaches beyond and propels into the future, i.e., cotranscends. The interrelational movement of the environment with the universe is such that negentropic energy interchange both enables and limits becoming.

Health

That health is defined as a process and not a state at a particular point in time is consistent with the other elements of Parse's model. Perception of health is recognized as unique to the person at the same time that it is being cocreated through the person's relationships with others. The fundamental place of personal and cultural values in determining one's health is clearly stated: "Health is man's style of living chosen ideals ... a synthesis of man's values selected from multidimensional experiences created in open energy interchanges with the environment" (Parse, p 31, 1981a). Patterns of relating value priorities constitute the person's health. The idea of transcending is stated in relation to health as the reaching beyond the actual to the possible through energy interchanges which occur between person and person, and person and environment. Coexistence as related to health involves risking of self and confrontation with the other, a synergistic rhythm leading toward more complex possibles and greater diversity. One pattern of the person's interrelationship with the world is disease. Hence, in this model health illness is not seen as a continuum, rather disease is suggested to be one possible universe of many in the person's environment. That is, disease could be viewed as in part one outcome of the choices and possibles resulting from man's open rhythmic energy exchange with the environment, one of those she/he may not know but is responsible for when making decisions.

Description of Nursing Activity

For Parse, the goal of nursing is "guiding the person and family in choosing among possibilities in the changing health process" (Parse, p 14, 1981a). Since one's perspective of health can be known only through a personal description, the nurse guides its sharing in the intersubjective relationship with the person and family. The meaning of the person's valuing and perspective of health is "expressed through patterns of relating the symbols of words, through tonality, tempo and volume, as well as gesture, gaze, touch and posture" (Parse, p 47, 1981a). The key to the elicitation of full and rich description is the "true presence of the nurse in the relationship" (Parse, p 54, 1981a). Relative to his/her/ their participation in the health experience, nurse and person or family seek to explore the possibles of the situation in order to choose the preferred way of being and becoming, to transform it into a new actual. The preferred nursing activity of this model then is communication, which can take place on many levels. For some nurses, the apparent lack of acknowledgement of nursing activity other than that carried through in the nurse-client interaction is inconsistent with caring for holistic man.

Interrelationships Among The Concepts

The interrelationships among the concepts of person, environment, health, and nursing may be expressed as follows: Nursing's focus is the person as a living unity, and directed toward guiding persons and families to participate in their health care. The person's behavior is multidimensional in structure and meaning. In the process of being and becoming over time, the person transcends her/his relative present in mutual simultaneous energy interchanges with the environment. Health is a continuously changing process of becoming uniquely perceived by the person, and cocreated through the person's interchange of energy with others and the environment. The person and her/his environment are expressions of pattern and organization of their interrelated energy fields in space-time. Disease is one expression of the person's interrelationship with the world. Nursing practice is directed toward illuminating and mobilizing persons' energies in light of lived values evidenced in their patterns of relating. The specific nature of nursing interventions, while creative and innovative, is rooted in the person's freedom to choose and responsibility for outcomes of all decisions.

Descriptions of Basic Concepts

The basic concepts of the model have been synthesized and deduced from the tenets, principles, and concepts from Rogers and the existential-phenomenological philosophers described in the above analysis. It is evident in Parse's elaboration of the meaning of the concepts that their derivation is primarily from the philosophical sources, and secondarily from the Rogers model. As will be seen, her syntheses are generally consistent with their origins.

There are nine concepts in the Parse model: 1) imaging; 2) valuing; 3) languaging; 4) revealing-concealing; 5) enabling-limiting; 6) connecting-separating; 7) powering; 8) originating; and, 9) transforming. Their explications demonstrate the phenomenological method: "a careful description of things as they appear and of the consciousness in which they appear" (Bannan, p 3, 1967). Kockelmans (1965) states further that "the object of phenomenological analysis and description consists in bringing to light those elements which initially are still hidden but in fact are ... the foundation of the immediately manifest traits of what shows itself to us" (p 22, 1965). To paraphrase and attempt to summarize the richness of meanings provided by Parse here, as in the discussion of the basic concepts, is the imposition of the logical analysis of parts on the phenomenological viewpoint of the whole.

Imaging is simultaneously giving form, structure, and meaning to prearticulate knowing. Meaning includes interpreting experiences encountered in the world and then according it significance in its incorporation into personal world view. It is a process reflective of the totality of the person. Valuing mirrors the person's world view (belief system) as it arises from interaction with the environment. This concept also draws on Raths, Merrill, and Simon's (1978) description of the valuing process. The key activities are choosing freely, prizing one's choices, and acting upon them.

The representation of one's structuring of reality is through languaging. Words as symbols are a function of cultural heritage, their meanings expressed all at once in interrelating through tonality, tempo, gesture, gaze, touch, and posture. The context of the situation in which languaging occurs affects its meaning. Revealing-concealing, enabling-limiting, connecting-separating, the next three concepts, are described as rhythmical patterns of Man-Living-Health. Their reasoning illustrates the dialectic method of juxtaposing opposed ideas and then resolving their conflict in a new unity. Revealing-concealing refers to the person's disclosing and not-disclosing in interaction with others, the coming to know oneself. In becoming, the person is enabled to move in one direction and limited in moving in another, i.e., the concept of enabling-limiting. Certain potentialities of the person are actualized at the same time as others are denied. Connecting-separating is described as a major mode of human development, each instance leading to a higher level of union. The separating of self from one phenomenon and connecting with another leads to integration of thought, greater complexity, and the seeking of new connections. Powering is seen as fundamental to being; it is the affirming of self in light of the potential of non-being. The rhythm of powering is the pushing-resisting which occurs in all relationships, and through tension and conflict creates possibles as one is present in the world. It is the essence of transcending, an essential part of human nature (Kockelmans, 1965). In distinguishing oneself from others, one originates a unique way of living the mutual energy interchange with environment. Originating is thus "the paradox of conforming-nonconforming certainty-uncertainty all at once" (Parse, p 60, 1981a). Transforming is the person's deliberate experience of struggling with change, continuous unfolding toward greater complexity. It is discovering new perspectives of self and others and from them forming new structures of meaning.

Relationships of Basic Concepts to Person, Health, Environment, Nursing

Parse's carefully outlined relationship of her basic concepts to nursing's general paradigm can be briefly stated as follows: From existential-phenomenological, philosophical, and Rogerian concepts and principles, nine concepts describing the person's interrelatedness with environment in becoming a person, as manifested in the continuously changing health process, have been deduced. She succinctly states the relationships among the derived concepts as:

Powering is a way of revealing and concealing imaging.

Originating is a manifestation of enabling and limiting valuing.

Transforming unfolds in the language of connecting and separating (Parse, p 69, 1981a).

As the nurse is inseparable from the person's being and becoming in the professional intersubjective relationship (environment), all of the basic and derived concepts are qually applicable to her/him in the process of nursing. Thus, the person and the nurse cocreate health in the environment in which they find themselves in the world. In Hardy's (1974) description of the syntax of theory, the relationships among all the concepts would be termed probabilistic.

INTERNAL ANALYSIS

Underlying Assumptions

Assumptions are untestable, formulated in terms of the theorist's perception of the world. While Parse notes that the model as a whole originates from lived nursing experience, the assumptions on which it is premised are explicitly specified, and their derivation from Rogers' model and philosophical sources is clear. Each of the seven foundational concepts is linked in at least one way with each of the others in the assumptions. As well, each assumption connects three of her derived concepts. Their relationship to Rogers' five assumptions is also evident, particularly with Rogers' first, fourth, and fifth, which reflect the latter's review of the philosophical literature. The assumptions are:

1. Man is coexisting while coconstituting rhythmical patterns with the environment.
2. Man is an open being, freely choosing meaning in situations, bearing responsibility for decisions.
3. Man is a living unity continuously coconstituting patterns of relating.
4. Man is transcending multidimensionally with the possibles.
5. Health is an open process of becoming experienced by man.
6. Health is a rhythmically coconstituting process of the man-environment relationship.
7. Health is man's patterns of relating value priorities.
8. Health is an intersubjective process of transcending with the possibles.
9. Health is unitary man's negentropic unfolding (Parse, p 25, 1981a).

The assumptions in the main reflect Parse's belief that nursing is rooted in the human sciences and is concerned with the person's unitary nature and qualitative experiences of health. Assumptions that man is an open system and an energy field which varies continuously can be considered implicit in 1, 5, and 9. Whether or not increasing complexity is seen as healthful cannot be interred from 4 and 9, particularly when, as noted earlier, disease is one pattern of relating with the environment. A belief that man's existence is his consciousness, the free and finite giving of meaning, and not a thing apart from consciousness (Bannan, 1967) is evident in 2 and 4. The existentialist tenet that transcendence is essential in man's nature is seen in 4 also.

Parse subscribes to the belief that the person is not a sum of the parts but rather is a unified being. Her conception of the human sciences as inclusive of all that are interconnected with man (1982) needs to be carefully distinguished from a generally understood definition of the human sciences as encompassing the humanities and social sciences only. Ellis (1968) notes that "ideally, theories most important for nursing would be those that encompass both biological and behavioral observations and have potential for explaining their relationships (p 219, 1968). However, the relevance of quantitative knowledge to the understanding of the person's being and becoming in Parse's theory is not clear. This may be because she accepts the existentialist-phenomenological belief in body as subject rather than object (Bannan, 1967), and/or because the differentiating of quantitative and qualitative knowledge of the person is a reductionist rather than a holistic approach to nursing in her view.

Central Components of the Model

The central components of the model Man-Living-Health are the nine concepts and their derived principles and theoretical structures. None of these components are descriptive of nursing per se, but rather relate to the phenomena of the person and her/his health, the stated rationale for the existence of nursing as a profession. Given this belief, Parse's approach to nursing theory development is understandable.

One can make the conjecture that Man-Living-Health as presented in Table 16.1 can be treated as a construct and therefore a component because Parse states "the structuring of the words ... with the hyphen demonstrate a conceptual bond among the words that creates a unity of meaning different from the individual words as they stand alone" (Parse, p 39, 1981a). This parallels both Kaplan's (1964) definition of a construct as conveying more meaning than the individual concepts separately and Dubin's definition of a summative unit as "having a property that derives from interrelations among other properties" (p 66, 1978). Kaplan further states that constructs are defined on the basis of observables. Though "living health" is cocreated through interrelationship with others, one's perspective of it is known through personal description. There are known cultural norms of behavior which can be observed in the person's unique ways of relating, and the person can provide subjective data of her/his health. When intersubjective and subjective data are considered in a holistic way, the construct/model Man-Living-Health becomes a way of explaining the empirical events of the person's being and becoming. A major difficulty in understanding and applying Parse's model is her position that the manifestations of Man-Living-Health cannot be dichotomized in any way. Dubin (1978) points out that the person's capacities as an observer, recorder, and retainer of complex phenomena coming within range of her/his sensory fields are such that one is not capable of seeing things whole.

Parse's model connects the basic concepts. The difficulty in analyzing this model lies in attempting to fit concepts described according to the phenomenological method to categories developed according to the logical method. Each of Parse's concepts denotes a process. Thus, they could be said to fall under Dubin's category of relational unit. However, in trying to demonstrate the relation, one is faced with sorting out from among the multiplicity of properties described as characteristic of the thing, the process, a specific relationship.

Principles in nursing have been equated with scientific laws and theories, indicating that principles may be translated from postulates, concepts, and the data (Hardy, 1974; Jacox, 1974). It is from this usage that Parse appears to be operating in her principle statements.

Principle 1. Structuring meaning multidimensionally is cocreating reality through the languaging of valuing and imaging (Parse, p 42, 1981a).

Principle 2. Cocreating rhythmical patterns of relating is living the paradoxical unity of revealing-concealing and enabling-limiting while connecting-separating (Parse, p 50, 1981a).

Table 16.1
The Theory of Man-Living Health

Assumptions

1. Man is coexisting while coconstituting rhythmical patterns with the environment.
2. Man is an open being, freely choosing meaning in situation, bearing responsibility for decisions.
3. Man is a living unity continuously coconstituting patterns of relating.
4. Man is transcending multidimensionally with the possibles.
5. Health is an open process of becoming, experienced by man.
6. Health is a rhythmically coconstituting process of the man-environment interrelationship.
7. Health is man's patterns of relating value priorities.
8. Health is an intersubjective process of transcending with the possibles.
9. Health is unitary man's negentropic unfolding.

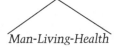

Man-Living-Health

Principles	Structuring meaning multi-dimensionally	Cocreating rhythmical patterns of relating	Cotranscending with the possibles
Concepts	Imaging Valuing Languaging	Revealing-concealing Enabling-limiting Connecting-separating	Powering Originating Transforming

Theoretical Structures   *Powering* is a way of *revealing and concealing imaging.*
Originating is a manifestation of *enabling and limiting valuing.*
Transforming unfolds in the *languaging of connecting and separating.*

(Reprinted with permission from Parse RR: Man-Living-Health: A Theory of Nursing. John Wiley & Sons Co., Inc., New York, 1981)

Principle 3.   Cotranscending with the possibles is powering unique ways of originating in the process of transforming (Parse, p 55, 1981a).

As statements of process, Parse's principles 2 and 3 meet this criterion of a time dimension necessary for a sequential law of interaction. Principle 1, however, is a categoric law of interaction (Dubin, 1978). Parse further elaborates the model in three statements which she calls theoretical structures. Each incorporates three of the concepts in a unique fashion related to the principles:

> Powering is a way of revealing and concealing imaging.
>
> Originating is a manifestation of enabling and limiting valuing.
>
> Transforming unfolds in the language of connecting and separating (Parse, p 69, 1981a).

These process statements cannot be considered propositions because they are not predictive values of the units. They do conform to Dubin's definition of law of interaction where it is the relationship, not the identified units, that is the lawful part of each statement. For example, the interaction in the third statement is "unfolds." These statements too may be classified as sequential laws of interaction because their units are not interchangeable as in a categoric law, and because of the temporal nature of process.

Relative Importance of The Components

The intricate interrelationships of language in the concepts, principles, and theoretical structures of this model make it difficult to assign their relative importance. This is consistent with its philosophical origins. The construct/model Man-Living-Health would appear to be the most important, with the identified concepts next in importance, as they are integral units of the principles intended to guide practice. The theoretical structures, to be verified in practice, then follow.

The individuality of the person is her/his behavior in choosing ways of living health. Viewing the person as an open system among other open systems, as does Rogers, and open to the world in Heidegger's terms (Kockelmans, 1965), leads to the incorporation of the concepts of powering, connecting-separating, enabling-limiting, and transforming. These build on mutual simultaneous energy interchange and negentrophy. This then allows for seeing the person, in choosing health values, becoming increasingly diverse and complex in her/his patterns of relating.

The patterns also evolve through the concepts of languaging and revealing-concealing. The concepts of imaging and originating demonstrate that the predictability of the person or family is through pattern and organization. The evolutionary perspective allows for change in the process of unfolding. Nursing intervention is concerned with consideration of these concepts as formulated in the principles and theoretical structures in assisting persons and families to choose among alternatives in the health process.

Relationships Among the Components

Specifying interactions is an indispensable part of model building (Hardy, 1974). Parse has clearly outlined the relationship and direction of components of her model.

The efficiency of laws of interaction is linked by Dubin (1978) to the range of units or concepts to which they apply. A law is of low efficiency when the range of variability in the values of the unit is broad. That all of the principles relate to the person is specified in the elaboration of their meaning, although the word "person" is not included in their definitions, and each indicates concurrent presence of the units. Thus Parse's principles in this way fit Dubin's categorization of laws of a low level of efficiency. However, he notes that the use of such laws may be a strategy of building theory to improve understanding of the phenomenon. The theoretical structures derived from the concepts and principles, also laws of interaction, further clarify the order of relationship among the units of the model. A theoretical structure is defined by Parse as "a statement of interrelating concepts in a way that can be verified" (Parse, p 68, 1981a). Given that the concepts are defined as processes, and are the units making up the structures, one can see that identification of suitable empirical indicators for verification constitutes a challenge.

Analysis of Consistency

Examination of the relationships among the components of Parse's model demonstrates the absence of internal self-contradiction and therefore the presence of consistency. The multiplicity of meanings to the elaborated structure of the concepts, principles, and theoretical structures is consistent with the phenomenological method of describing reality used in their development. Each assumption and each principle connects three of the deduced concepts, and the seven foundational concepts are related with each other at least once in the assumptions. One can then infer that all of the concepts are essential to the development of the model. The relative centrality of the person living health is clear, and the implications of changing a given principle, such as making meaning unidimensional rather than multidimensional is also clear. However, derivation of propositions from the principles to further explicate the relationships among the concepts is essential to provide adequate measures of their values (Dubin, 1978). Their absence at this point in the model's development may be related to Parse's view of person as unitary in nature, and the difficulty of empirically demonstrating synergistic behavior in measurable units.

Analysis of Adequacy

As the purpose of a scientific theory is to describe, explain, and predict a part of the empirical world (Hardy, 1974), its value in part lies in its adequacy in explaining and predicting the phenomena with which it is concerned. Suggested assessment criteria are scope, complexity, testability, usefulness, value explicitness, ability to generate information, and terminology (Ellis, 1968).

Parse's model orders observations about a variety of phenomena related to the person, encompassing behavioral manifestations, observations of the person's relating to self, others and the environment. While she states that all lived experiences are relevant, reference is not made to biological manifestations of the person in his/her being and becoming, nor to man collectively. The scope of nursing practice based on this model then appears to be limited in this aspect. As Ellis states, "scope should be judged in terms of the generalizations and phenomena pertinent to an individual . . . in circumstances which cause him to be labelled . . . patient" (p 219, 1968). Wellness care and mental health psychiatric care are areas of practice which clearly fit with this model. There is no doubt that the model has complexity, i.e., a multiplicity of variables and relationships as well as multiplicity of meaning to each of the units.

Both Dubin (1978) and Ellis (1968) state that testability is a significant criterion of theory adequacy. To be testable, one must be able to infer from the theory predictions which can be found to hold or not to hold. In this model, it appears difficult to develop the necessary rigorous linkage statements to be able to follow from observations and descriptions of reality to propositions and hypotheses. Propositions need to be developed to make the model a complete theoretical system. This is partly related to terminology. Kockelmans (1965) notes that to reduce the cultural world to the 'lived world,' one is almost forced to develop new terminology. However, it is important that the scientific language of a discipline be understood by its members. The ideas are abstract and highly philosophical, and their intersubjectivity of meaning, cited by Hardy as important for application, is likely to be clearer to philosophers than nurse scientists.

The difficulty in terminology also affects the fit of the model with practice. The novel usage of commonly understood words, and the construction of new words, e.g., cotranscending, could be difficult to relate to the generally understood concepts and terms about the person, family, and environment. The illustrative examples in the text are very useful in this regard, and do clarify the model's intents. The multiplicity of meanings is a strength in regard to the range of possible nursing interventions. However, the language and multiplicity of meanings leave the concepts open to confused use. A major strength of the model is its value explicitness presented in the assumptions and the concept valuing. The person's responsibility for choice and participation in the health process is clear.

EXTERNAL ANALYSIS

Relationship to Nursing Research

The major area of theory testing in research should be directed toward validating the relationships among theory components. The analysis of this model from the rigorous logical framework for theory construction outlined by Dubin and Hardy suggests there would be difficulties in its verification by use of the scientific method. Parse states her expectation that the model will be verified by descriptive methodologies. Her current research uses the phenomenological method in analyzing the meaning of health as a lived experience. Descriptions by 50 adult subjects of feeling healthy have been analyzed, and preliminary findings indicate that this approach is revealing a different conceptualization of health than the definitions currently found in the nursing literature (Parse, 1981b). Future studies will similarly analyze examples collected from other age groups (Parse, 1982).

In an emerging discipline such as nursing, an overemphasis on the scientific method may constrict rather than liberate its growth. Silva (1977) states that meaningfulness can be sacrificed for rigor in research, resulting in statistically significant findings with little value for clinical application. She argues the case for complementary methods to the scientific to derive nursing knowledge. Glaser and Strauss (1967) support her contention that an appropriate method for theory building is introspection, reflections on experience, one's own and others. This is congruent with the phenomenological method's purpose of describing and elucidating the meaning and structure of experience.

With this model, formulation of the necessary empirical generalizations to predict outcomes of prospective studies presents a challenge to the nurse researcher. This model has the potential to expand the descriptive base of nursing in regard to beliefs, behaviors, and their perceived meanings in life situations affecting health. An holistic approach to health care, and rising consumer expectations regarding health care services per se increases nursing's need to generate a more extensive knowledge base about the health process.

Parse suggests a number of situations appropriate to her model for investigation. For example:

Theoretical structure: Powering is a way of revealing and concealing imaging.

Lived experience	*Description*
Struggling with uncovering the hidden meaning in a dialogue.	Describe a situation in which you experienced yourself struggling to clarify the ambiguous messages in a conversation (Parse, p 79, 1981a).

Relationship to Nursing Education

A substantive knowledge base is essential for professional nursing practice. The generic program demands a solid base in both sciences and the humanities for the nursing component, while specialization at the graduate level provides increased depth in a particular area. Parse presents a comprehensive curriculum plan implementing her model at the graduate level. It is an excellent example of the application of curriculum and evaluation principles, demonstrating how to integrate a particular nursing model throughout all aspects of a program. As to be expected, the curriculum design is process oriented. Appropriately, the chosen field of specialization is family health. Given the existentialist-phenomenological foundation of the model, one would expect inclusion of a suitable philosophy course for supporting content. This would facilitate student understanding of the conceptual framework, as not all undergraduate programs have a philosophy requirement. The specific emphasis given to student learning in the area of theory development provides for knowledgeable users of theories in practice. The design of student learning experiences provides opportunities both for further elaboration of the model and confirmation of its usefulness for practice.

Relationship to Professional Nursing Practice

Parse's model would be an appropriate base for practice in any situation where the focus is on the person's communicative interaction with the nurse. Basing care planning on the client's perspective of health and her/his care would encourage innovation in activities designated nursing, and acceptance of unique self-care activities. In the example of a family situation described by Parse, the family's exploration of the meaning of the diagnosis of possible malignancy, care planning based on the three theoretical structures is discussed. For example, the nurse would focus on guiding the family in living with ambiguity (originating), to focus on resultant value changes (valuing), and to change health priorities (enabling-limiting). The specific interventions relevant to goals would be derived from the description of the impact of the diagnosis on each family member's health perspective as well as that on the family as a whole. Recognition of change in the person-family-environment mutual energy interchange is an integral part of the nursing process. One aspect of nursing's responsibility using this model is to assist the person to originate patterns of living coordinate with environmental patterns rather than in conflict. This requires concern for the multiplicity of events making up the universes of the person's environment. Data for the client profile would be qualitatively more detailed, with the likely outcome of greater specificity and flexibility in short and long range goals and a greater range of interventions. Given nursing's responsibility to guide the person and family in choices in the health process, with openness to change valued, Parse's model suggests greater creativity in the exploration of potentials for health. Accepting self and client as cocreating and cotranscending the environment implies the nurse's expectation of personal as well as professional change in her/his interaction with clients.

SUMMARY

Science has two directions: one towards abstractions-laws, unity, parsimony, integration; but also one towards comprehensiveness, the acceptance and description of all that exists (Maslow, 1966). Fitting the latter direction, Parse's model is quite different from other nursing models in the nature of its synthesis of concepts and principles from the disciplines of nursing and philosophy. As described, it also fits today's generally accepted nursing paradigm. It is a creative example of a model built according to the logical rules of theory building while maintaining the integrity of the phenomenological method of description. Parse has given us a commendable demonstration, particularly for nursing education, of her model's application in research, practice, and education. She notes that it is a theory in evolution, as are all theories. Its testing and use will determine its place in the development of nursing theory.

REFERENCES

Bannan JF: The Philosophy of Merleau-Ponty. Harcourt, Brace & World, Inc., New York, 1967

Barrett W: What is Existentialism? Grove Press, Inc., New York, 1964

Dubin R: Theory Building. The Free Press, New York, 1978

Ellis R: Characteristics of significant nursing theories. Nursing Research, Vol 17, No 3, pp 217-222, 1968

Glaser RG, Strauss A: The Discovery of Grounded Theory. Aldine Publishing Co., New York, 1967

Hardy MD: Theories: Components, development, evaluation. Nursing Research, Vol 23, No 2, pp 100-107, 1974

Jacox A: Theory construction in nursing: An overview. Nursing Research, Vol 17, No 3, pp 206-209, 1974

Kaplan A: The Conduct of Inquiry. Chandler Publishing Co., San Francisco, California, 1964

Kockelmans JJ: Martin Heidegger: A First Introduction to His Philosophy. Duquesne University Press, Pittsburgh, Pennsylvania, 1965

Maslow A: The Psychology of Science. Henry Regnery Co., Chicago, Illinois, 1966

Parse RR: Nursing Fundamentals. Medical Examination Publishing Inc., Flushing, New York, 1974

Parse RR: Man-Living-Health: A Theory of Nursing. John Wiley & Sons, Inc., New York, 1981a

Parse RR: Personal communication, December 18, 1981b

Parse RR: Paper presented at meeting of Sigma Theta Tau, Lambda Chapter, Detroit, Michigan, April 1982

Raths L, Harmin M, Simon S: Values and Teaching. Charles E. Merrill, Columbus, Georgia, 1978

Rogers M: An Introduction to the Theoretical Basis for Nursing. F.A. Davis Co., Philadelphia, Pennsylvania, 1970

Rogers M: Nursing: A science of unitary man. In Riehl J, Roy C (eds): Conceptual Models for Nursing Practice, 2nd ed, Appleton-Century-Crofts, New York, 1980

Silva MC: Philosophy, science, theory: Interrelationships and implications for nursing research. Image, Vol 9, pp 59-63, 1977

17

A LIFE PERSPECTIVE
RHYTHM MODEL

Joyce J. Fitzpatrick

Development of this conceptualization grew from a professional interest in how nurses can help people live through, move through, and grow and learn through, crisis experiences. More philosophically, this interest is in the meanings that persons attach to life—meanings that serve not only to enhance life but meanings which are essential to maintain life. Those who have no meaning do not continue to live. Understanding the essence of life's meaning refers not only to death by suicide but of all deaths—those who have lost the will to live, those who die having accomplished their life's purpose, and those who continuously court death, through high risk-taking behaviors to indirect self-destructive behaviors (e.g., diabetics who fail to take their insulin, heavy smokers, and alcohol and drug dependent persons). It seems as if the meaning attached to life is intimately linked to health, no matter whether health is defined as absence of disease, quality of life, or maximum wellness.

A review of the factors related to the experience and outcome of crisis situations led to the hypothesis that individuals experiencing crisis had difficulty integrating the present situation within their life perspective. This is consistent with clinical observations that individuals in crisis are very focused on the here and now, the current stressors, and the present experience. For example, the adolescent, experiencing a normal developmental crisis, is often described as desiring immediate satisfaction of present needs, of being unable to delay gratification, in short, of being focused on the here and now. Thus, knowledge of the crisis perspective and of developmental theories has been integrated within a nursing framework.

Within the crisis perspective there is the theoretical postulation that peak periods or sudden turning points could be identified within the human experience. The life process includes a series of crisis experiences which may be either developmentally or situationally initiated. Within a crisis experience there is both a threat to the integrity of the person and an opportunity for growth. A crisis is by definition time limited and represents a transitional phase in the person's experience of life (Fitzpatrick, 1982). One thing that is indeed heartening about crisis experiences is that they *do* end! There is no such thing as a constant crisis, a fact that can be most helpful in therapeutic intervention with individuals in crisis. Specific patterns have been identified which characterize the crisis experience where crisis experiences are conceptualized within the rhythm perspective (i.e., it is assumed that the rhythm of life is manifested through crises). Life's crisis experiences represent the rhythmic peaks in the human developmental process. This conceptualization led to the identification of possible indices of human functioning. Those that are proposed include temporal patterns, motion patterns, consciousness patterns, and perceptual patterns as characteristics of humans (Fitzpatrick, 1980).

SUMMARY OF EMPIRICAL FINDINGS

During this period of developing conceptualizations about the human experience of life, and thus health, my empirical investigations have been primarily focused on the descriptions of temporal patterns, with some additional focus on the other identified patterns. More recently, the research has directly addressed the meanings of death and, thus, the meanings of life. This recent research on life and death stems not only from the basic concern but also from the empirical investigations on patterns of human functioning. Specifically, the more general problem of the meaning of life has been rediscovered through the specific research on time and has directly led to the conceptual development of this life perspective rhythm model.

In the initial study, the research was focused on the way in which healthy individuals related their subjective temporal pattern to that of the environment (Fitzpatrick, 1975). The basic theoretical postulation was that persons who were focused on the present would be very much aware of the passage of time. An underlying theoretical postulation was that mentally healthy persons accurately perceived their environment and, in fact, their focus on the present was important to their mental health. It is generally accepted that mentally healthy, reasonable persons get places on time. Somehow these persons have control over their lives and, thus, control of time.

In retrospect, the major contribution of the study seems to be that it generated questions not only about the conceptualizations but also about the measurement of the experience of time. The study seemed to represent a traditional linear view of temporal patterns and of health. Following this investigation, it seemed necessary to directly attend to the multidimensional nature of human experience.

Two studies were then designed with significant attempts to study temporal and motor patterns from the crisis perspective. It was argued that the crisis and experience of institutionalization, nursing home residence and hospitalization, would lead to identification of differences between groups on the basis of environmental situation.

The first of these studies, that of nursing home residents, (Fitzpatrick and Donovan, 1978), was of particular importance in the design of future research. Clearly, the noninstitutionalized elderly persons were more present oriented than the institutionalized elderly persons—a fact that they attributed to their necessary and continual attention to present crises or potential crises. They generally described themselves as having to focus on the here and now in order to remain in control of their lives. The institutionalized elderly persons described themselves as having little control over their own experience. Their lives were planned for them. This study focused on comparisons between older and younger persons, the beginning of research with a developmental orientation. Clear distinctions on the basis of developmental stage have emerged through the series of investigations (Donovan, Fitzpatrick, and Johnston, 1980a; 1981; Fitzpatrick and Donovan, 1978; Johnston, Fitzpatrick, and Donovan, 1981).

The study of hospitalized individuals was another focus on the environmental situation as related to temporal experiencing (Fitzpatrick, Johnston, and Donovan, 1980b). The hospitalized group was more past and present oriented, with even the past focus being related to the period immediately preceding hospitalization. So in a sense, these persons could be understood as focusing on the present crisis. It was also interesting to note that time passed slowly for these hospitalized persons, a characteristic which is also directly linked to the crisis experience. Individuals in crisis generally think that there is no end, that time is passing slowly (Fitzpatrick, Johnston, Donovan, 1980a).

Following these studies, specific questions were raised about temporal experiencing within crisis situations. A series of studies among death-involved individuals was planned. It was reasoned that the crisis of dying represented the most complex and differentiated phase of a person's growth. Thus, it was anticipated that the behavioral manifestation related to temporal patterns characterizing this developmental phase would be that of a sense of timelessness. Again the hypothesis was consistent with clinical observations of dying persons, with whom time as linear reality has no meaning, yet time as subjective reality is all meaningful (Fitzpatrick, 1980).

Three distinct death-involved groups have thus far been studied—terminally ill cancer patients cognizant of their terminal illness, suicidal individuals, and aged individuals. The underlying theoretical proposition regarding these clinical groups is that more similarities than differences would be identified in the various temporal dimensions in that (1) they are all experiencing a crisis, and (2) they are all intimately involved with death. Similarities have been identified with respect to some of the temporal dimensions. For example, the death-involved individuals have a limited future perspective and are focused more directly on the near past, the present, and the immediate future; and they generally report a heightened sense of time pressure. There is no clear indication from the data whether time passes slowly or quickly for them. The extent to which this reflects a sense of timelessness is yet to be evaluated. There does exist some support for the basic temporal components of crisis theory. For example, the time limited nature of the crisis is reflected in the focus on a brief future. The tendency to focus on the present situation is clearly expressed by the individuals in crisis (Fitzpatrick, 1980; Fitzpatrick, Donovan and Johnston, 1980a, 1980b).

The issues of paramount concern which have been generated through the series of studies have to do with conceptualization and measurement of temporality, or temporal patterns, which characterize life's rhythm. While the research related to rhythms, particularly biological and circadian rhythms, is extensive, it is also apparent that the conceptualizations underlying these investigations are contiguous rather than comparable and exact in reference to human rhythms. The task remains to continue to describe the temporal rhythm patterns throughout the developmental process and during crisis experiences. Some tentative statements have emerged from this research. Some of these statements are more generally related to overall research on rhythmic phenomena, some are related more specifically to the developmental crisis of dying, and some provide strong hints of intervention strategies for persons in crisis. Specific attention to each of these areas would seem to be most advantageous in the future advancement of scientific discoveries.

PROPOSAL OF A LIFE PERSPECTIVE MODEL

As a result of this theoretical and empirical study, a life perspective rhythm paradigm is proposed. This conceptualization not only offers an organizing and integrating framework for research on human rhythms but also provides a variety of avenues for significant research related to health. For example, differences identified in rhythmic patterns of persons with varying health patterns would be most relevant to this conceptualization. Consistencies between the environmental rhythms such as light, dark and the human rhythms of sleep, wake, emotions and moods, pain, and level of consciousness or mental alertness would be explored. These examples provide some beginning pathways for further scientific conjectures regarding the phenomena of nursing's concern.

This life perspective rhythm model is based on the conceptualizations of unitary man proposed by Rogers (1970, 1980). The basic assumptions proposed by Rogers and the principles upon which Rogers' model is based are central to this developing life perspective model. Rogers' assumptions include:

1. Man is a unified whole possessing his own integrity and manifesting characteristics that are more than and different from the sum of his parts;
2. Man and environment are open systems, continually exchanging matter and energy with each other;
3. The life process evolves irreversibly and unidirectionally along the space time continuum;
4. Pattern and organization identify man and reflect his innovative wholeness;

5. Man is characterized by the capacity for abstraction and imagery, language and thought, sensation and emotion (Rogers, 1970).

Rogers' principles focus on man and environment as open systems, and further describe the changes that characterize the evolutionary development of man and environment. These principles include:

1. *Helicy* which describes the nature and direction of change as continuously innovative, probabilistic, and characterized by increasing complexity and diversity of field pattern and organization emerging from their continuous interaction and manifesting nonrepeating rhythmicities.
2. *Resonancy* which describes the human field and enviromental field as identified by wave pattern and organization manifesting changes from lower frequency, longer waves to higher frequency, shorter waves.
3. *Complementarity* which describes the process of continuous mutual interaction between human and environmental fields (Rogers, 1980).

This life perspective rhythm model is a developmental model which proposes that the process of human development is characterized by rhythms. Human development occurs within the context of continuous person/environment interaction. Basic human rhythms that describe the development of persons include the identified indices of holistic human functioning, i.e., temporal patterns, motion patterns, conciousness patterns, and perceptual patterns. The rhythmic correlates developed by Rogers are consistent with this life perspective rhythm model. Human development is understood to proceed rhythmically. Throughout the developmental process one can identify peaks and troughs of particular human rhythms with the overall progression toward faster rhythms. For example, in relation to temporal patterns one can identify the basic progression of the rhythm as moving from time passing slowly, through time passing quickly, toward timelessness. While this describes the overall life pattern, from infancy through dying, it is also possible to identify and describe the changes *within* the overall life pattern. Thus, within one's life this overall pattern may continue an infinite number of times, with continuous progression toward timelessness becoming more dominant as development occurs. This may best be described as patterns within a pattern or rhythms within an overall life rhythm. While these indices of holistic human functioning can be described by their characteristics as rhythms, they can also be described by their relationship to health, where health is conceptualized as a basic human dimension. Thus, health is viewed as a continuously developing characteristic of humans with the full life potential that may characterize the process of dying—the heightened awareness of the meaningfulness of life—representing a more fully-developed dimension of health (humanness).

The life perspective is described by a dimension of health or humanness. The meaning attached to life, the basic understanding of human existence, is a central concern of nursing as science and profession.

Nursing interventions can be focused on enhancing the developmental process toward health so that individuals may be led to develop their potential as human beings. A range of possible intervention modalities can be explored for their effectiveness in enhancing health and development. At the same time, nursing science can be focused on the continuing exploration of proposed relationships among basic concepts of person and health, and the further delineation of the indices of holistic human functioning.

SUMMARY

It is recognized that what is proposed here is a brief sketch of the developing conceptualizations of human experience. Chapter 18 is an analysis of this conceptualization based on review of the empirical research and the theoretical bits and pieces that have been presented over the years as the conceptualization has developed. In all respects, this task is completed to communicate that this is now, that these current understandings may enhance the creative development of nursing science.

REFERENCES

Donovan MJ, Fitzpatrick JJ, Johnston RL: Temporal experiences related to the developmental process of aging. Paper presented at the American Psychological Association Convention, Montreal, Canada, September, 1980

Donovan MJ, Fitzpatrick JJ, Johnston RL: Aging, time, and health. Paper presented at the American Psychological Association Annual Convention, Los Angeles, California, August, 1981

Fitzpatrick JJ: An investigation of the relationship between temporal orientation, temporal extension, and time perception. Unpublished doctoral disseration, New York University, New York, 1975

Fitzpatrick JJ: Patients' perceptions of time: Current research. International Nursing Review, Vol 27, pp 148-153, 1980

Fitzpatrick JJ: The crisis perspective: Relationship to nursing. In Fitzpatrick JJ, Whall AL, Johnston RL, Floyd JA: Nursing Models and Their Psychiatric Mental Health Applications, Robert J Brady Co., Bowie, Maryland, 1982

Fitzpatrick JJ, Donovan MJ: Temporal experience and motor behavior among the aging. Research in Nursing and Health, Vol 1, pp 60-68, 1978

Fitzpatrick JJ, Donovan MJ, Johnston RL: Experience of time during the crisis of cancer. Cancer Nursing, Vol 3, pp 191-194, 1980a

Fitzpatrick JJ, Johnston RL, Donovan MJ: Hospitalization as a crisis: Relation to temporal experiences. Paper presented at The 13th Annual Conference of the Western Society for Research in Nursing, Los Angeles, California, April 30-May 2, 1980b

Johnston RL, Fitzpatrick JJ, Donovan MJ: Developmental stage: Relationship to temporal dimensions. Paper presented at the ANA Council of Nurse Researchers Annual Meeting, Washington, D.C., September, 1981

Rogers ME: An Introduction to the Theoretical Basis of Nursing. F.A. Davis Co., Philadelphia, Pennsylvania, 1970

Rogers ME: Nursing: A science of unitary man. In Riehl J, Roy C (eds): Conceptual Models for Nursing Practice, 2nd ed, Appleton-Century-Crofts, New York, 1980

18

FITZPATRICK'S RHYTHM MODEL: ANALYSIS FOR NURSING SCIENCE

Jana L. Pressler

Theoretical meaning evolves from the interaction of scientific content with critical review. To adequately assess the significance of proposed nursing models, the criteria used to judge scientific merit must be carefully selected. Equating the discipline of nursing with a community of scholars (Ellis, 1982a), evaluative components espoused by Ellis (1968), Hardy (1974, 1978), and Newman (1979) have been chosen as a logical foundation from which to analyze the emerging meaning of Fitzpatrick's life perspective rhythm model for nursing.

HISTORICAL EVOLUTION OF THE MODEL

Using an historical method, Fitzpatrick's (1983) life perspective rhythm model fits the description of a theoretical model. Fitzpatrick's first formal explanation of her nursing model was presented in a paper at the Indiana University School of Nursing in 1979 (Fitzpatrick, 1979). Before that time, Fitzpatrick's research and academic endeavors focused heavily on temporal and motion patterns with minimal mention or integration of consciousness or perceptual patterns.

A scatter diagram may be formulated by graphically plotting Fitzpatrick's scholarly work (see Figure 18.1). With time representing the x-axis and indices of human functioning as the y-axis, an illustration of the increasing complexity in number and kind of human patterns investigated is achieved. Flaherty and Fitzpatrick's (1978) study looking at a relaxation technique involving motion, consciousness, and perception appears to be the research triggering mechanism for Fitzpatrick's (1979) exposition of a theoretical model.

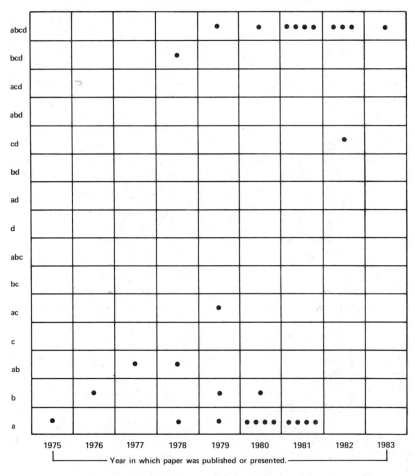

Indices of Wholistic Human Functioning
a - temporal patterns   c - consciousness patterns
b - motion patterns   d - perceptual patterns
● - represents the patterns which were addressed either singly or in combination over the years (reference citations for these years are listed in the reference section)

Figure 18.1. Fitzpatrick's Conceptual Movement Toward a Model for Nursing.

BASIC CONSIDERATIONS

An analysis of Fitzpatrick's rhythm model for nursing science begins with the distinctive way in which person, environment, health, and nursing are defined and related. These four elements are all intimately linked with meaning essential to life.

Fitzpatrick (1983) sees "meaning" as the most crucial portion of human experience. According to Fitzpatrick (1979, 1980, 1983), meaning is necessary to maintain and enhance life. Rogers' (1979) postulated correlates of human development are used as a basis for further ordering and explicating life's reality.

Rogers' (1979) correlates of shorter, higher frequency waves which manifest shorter rhythms and approach a seemingly continuous patterning serve as Fitzpatrick's foci for hypothesizing the existence of rhythmic patterns. Rogers' position that the human life span approximates transformation with human development aimed toward transcendence is incorporated within Fitzpatrick's quantitative and qualitative descriptions of life perspective. The developmental correlate whereby time seems timeless represents a beginning of Fitzpatrick's theorizing regarding temporal patterns. Motion patterns are similarly derived from Rogers' proposal of motion seeming to be continuous as development proceeds. Consciousness patterns are closely aligned with Rogers' idea that one progresses from sleeping to waking and to beyond waking. The correlates of "visibility" becoming more ethereal in nature and "heaviness" approaching a more weightless phase are the basis for Fitzpatrick's perceptual patterns.

Definitions of Person and Environment

Fitzpatrick's overall life perspective is synthesized from interpretations made from Rogers' (1979) developmental correlates. Envisioned as patterns within a pattern, or rhythms within a life rhythm (Fitzpatrick, 1983), Fitzpatrick's rhythm patterns are explicit operational modes which specify the pattern of person and environment explicated by Rogers (1980). Occurring within the context of rhythmical person/environment interaction, indices of holistic human functioning are identified by Fitzpatrick as temporal, motion, consciousness, and perceptual patterns (Fitzpatrick, 1979, 1980, 1982a, 1983). Fitzpatrick's writings are consistent with the Rogerian position regarding person and environment being open systems in continuous interaction.

Fitzpatrick (1983) asserts that the four indices of human functioning identified above are intricately related to health patterns throughout the life span. She also proposes that these indices can be described as rhythmic in nature. In a projection of Rogers' (1970, 1980) principle regarding the symphonic interaction of persons and their environments, Fitzpatrick (1982a) postulates the dynamic concepts of congruency, consistency, and integrity as complementary with rhythmic patterns. Attention to the nonlinear character of patterns supports Fitzpatrick's utilization of Rogers' (1980) specifications regarding four-dimensionality.

Definition of Health

Two distinct interpretations of Smith's (1981) clinical and eudaemonistic models of health illness are contained in Fitzpatrick's explanation of health. According to Fitzpatrick (1983), health shares the health interpretations of Smith (1981), i.e., absence of disease (clinical), quality of life, and maximum wellness (eudaemonistic). By themselves, gradations of the term "sick" are believed to be too eclectic to effectively embellish a definition of health (Fitzpatrick, 1981a). Instead, health is conceptualized as a basic human dimension which is undergoing continuous development. A more fully developed phase of human health is buttressed by an optimum life potential which might be exemplified through the process of dying or a heightened awareness of the meaningfulness of life.

Definition of Nursing

The ontogenetic and phylogenetic interactions among person and health are looked upon as the essence of nursing (Fitzpatrick, 1983). Fitzpatrick attends not only to relationships within or between these juxtaposed elements, and in so doing, includes latent relationships "outside" of person and health proper. Having the salient concern of these relationships as the meaning attached to life, nursing is understood to be a science worthy of professional status (Fitzpatrick, 1982c). Nursing interventions are perceived as facilitating the developmental process toward health.

An important clarification should be made regarding Fitzpatrick's usage of "perspective" in characterizing her model for nursing. More limited in scope than a "world view," the concept of perspective described by Fitzpatrick might be interchanged with the term "paradigm" or "paradigmatic view." As defined by Kuhn (1970), a paradigm represents a unique description of phenomena yet lacks a dramatically new world view. Paradigms usually have obvious associations with existing world views and share like orientations. Fitzpatrick's reliance on Rogers' (1970, 1980) five basic assumptions and homeodynamic principles substantiate a bond with an established world view for nursing.

Relationships Among Concepts

Person, environment, health, and nursing are all addressed in Fitzpatrick's theoretical model. Because person and environment are viewed as integral with one another and having no real boundaries, one can assume that environment is implied when the term person is used. Although Fitzpatrick (1983) does not go into great detail in outlining her perception of environment, her publications consistently mirror a basic Rogerian (1980) definition of environmental field. The human element is treated as an open, holistic, rhythmic system that can best be described by temporal, motion, consciousness, and perceptual patterns. Her four-fold entity of person is enhanced by awareness of the meaningfulness of life, or health. Greater than in meaning and different from an explanation of health itself, nursing's central concern is focused on person in relation to health. The relationships among all four elements are shown in Figure 18.2.

Figure 18.2 categorizes the essential theoretical elements of person, environment, health, nursing and nursing activity as if one were looking through a longitudinal beginning (or end) of a Slinky®. The Slinky® represents the life spiral. The science and art of nursing are specifically labelled as "nursing" and "nursing activity" respectively. Health is integrated within the overall life pattern in mutual interaction with person, environment, nursing, and nursing activity. The pendulum represents person's rhythmic patterns. Through the evolutionary movement of the basic model, a pendulum perspective of the rhythmic patterns of human functioning comes into view. A glimpse of the camouflaged Slinky® reappears through the vibrations emitted during pendular sway.

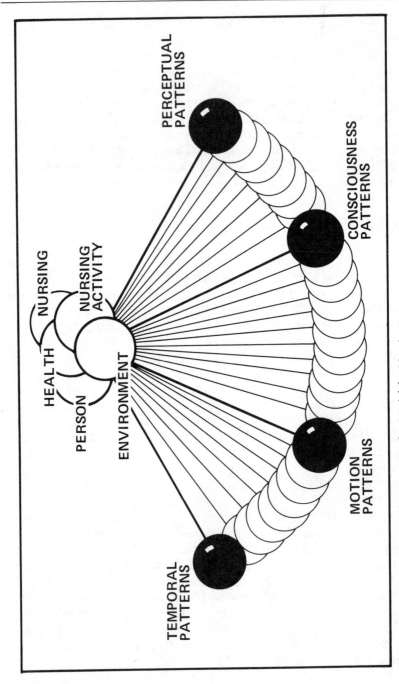

Figure 18.2. Relationships Within Fitzpatrick's Model for Nursing.

The permeating notions of acausality and curvilinear four-dimensionality found within Fitzpatrick's model make the task of placing her concepts in some linear format rather incongruous. Instead, the concepts are placed as reference points in the figure.

Knowing that Fitzpatrick has studied extensively with Rogers (and that Rogers uses a Slinky® to symbolize her world view of the science of unitary man) suggests the incorporation of a Slinky® in picturing some of the nonlinear relationships found within Fitzpatrick's model. A simplified rendition of Bentov's (1977) pendulum is employed in the representation of Fitzpatrick's (1983) rhythmic patterns of human functioning. Although the pendulum simulates linearity when viewed in rapid motion (refer to Fitzpatrick's [1980] discussion of a picket fence), it is purposely being used to depict nonlinear phenomena.

INTERNAL ANALYSIS

Fitzpatrick (1983) constructs her theoretical model with the help of conceptual underpinnings of Rogers' (1970, 1980). Rogers' (1970) five explicit assumptions about man as a unified whole, man and environment as open systems, the life process evolving irreversibly along space time, pattern and organization identifying man, and man as a sentient being, capable of abstraction, language, and thought provide a beginning framework for Fitzpatrick's basic considerations about person, environment, health, and nursing. Energy fields, openness, pattern and organization, and four-dimensionality (Rogers, 1980), along with Rogers' (1979) ten postulated correlates of human development further assist Fitzpatrick in proposing rhythmic patterns of holistic human functioning. Rogers' (1970, 1980) homeodynamic principles of helicy, resonancy, and complementarity reflect Fitzpatrick's basic beliefs regarding the evolutionary development of person and environment.

Several implicit assumptions pertinent to an understanding of Fitzpatrick's model were identified through an examination of prior writings. These include:

1. Differences in behavioral manifestations are more easily identified during the peaks of wave patterns (Fitzpatrick, p 153, 1980).

2. Identified by congruency, consistency, and integrity of rhythmic patterns, health is the manifestation of symphonic interaction of persons and their environments (Fitzpatrick, p 33, 1982a).

3. Emphasized through selected research on temporality, the meaning attached to life is a central concern of nursing (Fitzpatrick, 1981c).

4. Nursing is a philosophy, a science, and an art (Fitzpatrick, p 5, 1982c).

The central components of Fitzpatrick's model for nursing are distinguishable through the above assumptions. Person, environment, rhythmic patterns, the meaning attached to life, health, and nursing are all viewed essential in the life perspective rhythm model.

According to Hardy (1974), a first step in evaluating a theoretical premise is an appraisal of the validity of the assumptions, the validity of meanings attributed to the concepts, and the logic of the theoretical system. This kind of analytical sector allows for an overall assessment of meaning and logical adequacy.

The explicit Rogerian (1970) assumptions (regarding the essence of man and environment) postulated by Fitzpatrick are representative of a synthesis of a number of areas of knowledge. Clearly, Fitzpatrick's (1980) first implicit assumption about peaks of wave patterns is primarily derived from biological rhythm theory (Haus, 1964; Luce, 1970), and Caplan's (cited in Fitzpatrick, 1982a) interpretation of crisis theory. Fitzpatrick's (1982a) reformulation of the crisis perspective in relation to Rogers' (1970, 1979, 1980) conceptualizations relates to the second assumption concerning health. Similar to Rogers' (1970, 1980) approach, the concept of health is somewhat abstract. Health research which supports the existence of congruence, consistency, and integrity per se within Fitzpatrick's rhythmic patterns (described as peaks and troughs) of human functioning has yet to be documented. The concept of health as a critical component of the model warrants additional questioning and development as evidenced by:

1. Fitzpatrick (1983) entitles her model "A Life Perspective Rhythm Model" in lieu of "A Health Rhythm Model;"

2. The meaning attached to life is stated as being essential to life (Fitzpatrick, p 295, 1983) with secondary mention of health's importance;

3. Fitzpatrick (p 295, 1983) states, "Those who have no meaning do not continue to live" (she does not specify for those who have no health . . .); and

4. Her statement, "It seems as if the meaning attached to life is intimately linked to health . . ." (Fitzpatrick, p 295, 1983), is not a very stalwart introductory defense of health's reality.

Fitzpatrick has not directly laid claim to any of the implicit assumptions identified in this critique. Therefore, it is understandable that her conceptualization of health might be characterized somewhat differently in her model. However, the third assumption is supported by her past extensive work with temporality (Donovan et al., 1980, 1981; Fitzpatrick, 1975, 1977, 1980, 1981e, 1982a; Fitzpatrick & Donovan, 1978a, 1978b; Fitzpatrick et al., 1979, 1980; Johnston et al., 1981). Rogers' (1970) view of nursing is again visible within the final implicit assumption. As articulated by Fitzpatrick (1981b, 1982c), the broader dimensions of the profession of nursing can be characterized as philosophical, scientific, and artistic. These complementary nursing dimensions constitute an evolving theme in Fitzpatrick's work.

All of the explicit and implicit assumptions, except that of congruency, consistency, and integrity of human rhythmic patterns, seem clearly and logically defined within the model. If attention were given toward explaining what is meant by congruency, consistency, and integrity in patterns, these ideas would seem more plausible.

Brief theoretical descriptions for the elements of person, environment, health, nursing, and nursing activity are stated in Fitzpatrick's (1983) beginning sketch of the model. Of these five equally significant terms, the major discussion rests with person and health.

Rogerian explanations are used as Fitzpatrick's foundation for interpreting person and environment, even though Rogers' (1980) definitions of human field and environmental field are not presented in the model. According to Fitzpatrick, the human repertoire is further characterized by basic rhythms in the form of temporal patterns, motion patterns, consciousness patterns, and perceptual patterns. As stated earlier, ideas for these patterns were synthesized from Rogers' (1979) correlates of human development. All of the proposed patterns are equally important and at the same time different from each other. Perceptual patterns, however, are subsidiary to consciousness patterns. The notion of 'visibility' and 'heaviness' contained in perceptual patterns would logically fit within one's dimension of consciousness and, consequently, is redundant of consciousness. Newman's (1979) views about health would lead one to believe that temporal patterns and motion patterns might fall within an expanded pattern of consciousness.

According to Fitzpatrick (1983), health is closely affiliated with the meaning attached to life:

> It seems as if the meaning attached to life is intimately linked to health, no matter whether health is defined as absence of disease, quality of life, or maximum wellness (Fitzpatrick, p 295, 1983).

However, the words "no matter" make this statement a little confusing in determining how health is actually being conceptualized by Fitzpatrick. One interpretation might be that the meaning attached to life is intimately linked to health, regardless of how health is defined. Another possible explanation is that the meaning attached to life is intimately linked to health, with a notion of health including aspects of absence of disease, quality of life, or maximum wellness. Because she specifically gives three commonly-used descriptions of health, one might deductively select the latter understanding of health.

As a continuously developing characteristic of humans, or a basic human dimension, Fitzpatrick (1983) implies that health is in a perpetual phase of flux or rhythm. In a subsequent sentence, she contends that the development of health can be related to the full life potential, the process of dying, heightened awareness of the meaningfulness of life, and more fully-developed humanness.

Tillich (1961), in an article on the meaning of health, states that in order to speak of health, one must speak of all of the dimensions of life which are united in man. He points out that meanings are defined only by being brought into configuration with other meanings; hence, health is meaningful only in confrontation with its opposite. In her discussion about indices of holistic human functioning, Fitzpatrick suggests dimensions of human life which are united in person. Although she appears to be struggling with an operational definition of health, Fitzpatrick equates humanness with a dimension of health. She further states that a dimension of health describes the life perspective.

Utilizing the idea of ontogeny within phylogeny, the life perspective is also described as patterns within a pattern or rhythms within an overall life rhythm. She attends to the opposite of "the meaning of life" in asserting, "Those who have no meaning do not continue to live" (Fitzpatrick, p 295, 1983). With respect to Tillich's (1961) criteria, Fitzpatrick, therefore, satisfactorily speaks to a meaning of health. Even so, Fitzpatrick's (1976, 1981a, 1981c, 1982c) previous writings on health would lead one to think that her consideration of health has not yet reached its final form.

Two distinct definitions for nursing are given in Fitzpatrick's (1983) rhythm model. Nursing, as a noun, is described as the science and profession whose central concern is the meaning attached to life (health). As a verb, nursing is said to be focused on enhancing the developmental process toward health so that individuals may be led to develop their potentials as human beings. The way in which nursing as a philosophy fits in with these explanations of nursing is unclear in the 1983 publication. In an earlier work, Fitzpatrick (1982c) asserts that the ideals and truths embedded in the philosophy and science of nursing serve to guide professional practice. More detail regarding what is meant by "nursing philosophy" is still needed to demonstrate the usefulness of this concept for nursing.

Fitzpatrick (1982c) states that scientific inquiry is knowledge generation: knowledge which is applied in professional practice rather than a "practice theory" approach to the science of nursing. She states that because science and practice are complementary rather than similar, attempts to study the art of nursing will fall short. Unmistakably, then, nursing as a science is deemed precedent to nursing activity, according to Fitzpatrick. Although Rogers (1970) places scattering importance on health, Fitzpatrick's views of nursing generally concur with Rogers' portrayal of nursing as a basic science.

Fitzpatrick's supports the inclusion of philosophic ways of knowing in the development of science. She writes:

> Have we, in our quest for scientific and academic legitimacy and autonomous practice, lost sight of the philosophic basis of nursing? Science gives us knowledge but only philosophy can give us wisdom. . . . the art of nursing has its basis in both wisdom and knowledge, both philosophy and science. The ideals and truths inherent in the words love, courage, and honor serve to guide that

professional practice and at the same time attach meaning to the scientific understandings and applications
(Fitzpatrick, p 1, 1981b).

Fitzpatrick's explicit and implicit assumptions connect the
essential nursing concepts of person, environment, health and
nursing into a unified whole (refer to the prior discussion regarding the implicit assumption which looks at health). There is also a
consistent internal flow of ideas beginning with the assumptions
and proceeding to the derived nursing interventions. Occurring
within the context of an open, continuous person/environment
interaction, the life perspective rhythm model is specifically formulated as a developmental model.

EXTERNAL ANALYSIS

The extent to which a model is potentially useful to the profession is assessed in terms of external analysis. According to Ellis
(1968), the essential criticism of theoretical usefulness is use in
practice along with a careful observation of the results. Hardy
(1978) continues by reporting that theoretical ideas cannot be
empirically valid if they are logically inadequate. She also contends that empirical validity is perhaps the single most important
criterion for evaluating a theoretical tradition intended for later
application in a practice setting. Theoretical postulations must be
rigorously tested by empirical studies before they can be accepted
and actually utilized in nursing practice. Keeping these thoughts
in mind, one can begin looking at how Fitzpatrick, through
research activities, arrived at specific conceptualizations.
   A holistic approach to inquiry consists of the identification
of patterns which are reflective of the whole (Newman, 1979).
Newman (1979) asserts that this type of research methodology is
not to be confused with a complex, multivariate approach, nor the
summing up of many factors to make a whole.
   In order to include patterns of holistic human functioning in
a model, it is necessary to determine scientific ways for measur-
ing behaviors characteristic of the patterns, and relationships
among them. Because this is a cumbersome undertaking, no
direct testing of the basic relationships posited has been completed. Since, as a whole, the model is not operationally defined in
measurable terms, certainly the empirical adequacy of the
introductory perspective cannot be analyzed in any straightforward fashion. What follows is an overview of the empirical sup-

port that exists for including particular components in the model's theoretical claims.

Various kinds of support are suggested for the human rhythmic patterns of temporality, motion, consciousness, and perception from data housed in student research projects. Fitzpatrick's conceptualizations have been investigated by graduate students in nursing. Studies looking at temporality in combination with adult and elderly populations (Smokvina, 1976; Brasuell, 1977; Jones, 1977; Bouwman, 1979; Johnston, 1980; Kotal, 1980; Engle, 1981; Moore, 1981; Ramin, 1982; Schorr, 1982), temporality in association with psychiatric patients (Grider, 1977; Nalinnes, 1977; Mack, 1978; Chaffer, 1979; Alford, 1981), and temporality in relation to terminally ill individuals (Hartline, 1978) provide a workable base from which to establish the existence of temporal patterns. From a holistic perspective of life-span, however, Fitzpatrick lacks nursing research focused on infants', children's, and adolescents' notions of temporality.

Both younger and elderly groups have been addressed in investigating motion (Smokvina, 1976; Goldberg & Fitzpatrick, 1980; Roberts & Fitzpatrick, 1982; Sipols-Lenss, 1982). Nevertheless, patterns of consciousness have again been essentially examined in older age group contexts (Flaherty & Fitzpatrick, 1978; Jablonski, 1978; Pacini & Fitzpatrick, 1982; Roslaniec & Fitzpatrick, 1979; Floyd, 1982b; Horowitz, 1982).

Other types of perceptual patterns, i.e., perception of color (Fromme, 1979; McDonald, 1981) and music (Ludwig-Bonney, 1981) have been investigated. Because one's perception would seem to be dependent upon a present pattern of consciousness, these studies would relate to the patterns of consciousness.

Admitting that her investigative efforts have been primarily centered around temporal patterns, Fitzpatrick (1983) briefly summarizes some of the results which lend support to the theoretical model. She points out that in order to examine the meaning attached to life, it is critical for phenomena to be explored using a multidimensional approach.

Empirical support for the existence of nonlinear temporal patterns emerged from a number of research endeavors. Results from Fitzpatrick's 1975 study helped identify the need for generating questions about ways to measure the experience of time. The prevalence of temporal distinctions on the basis of differences in development were apparent in succeeding studies (Donovan et al., 1980; 1981; Fitzpatrick & Donovan, 1978;

Johnston et al., 1981). A sense of timelessness was described as being characteristic of behaviors identified among death-involved individuals (Fitzpatrick, 1980; Fitzpatrick, Donovan, & Johnston, 1980; Fitzpatrick, Johnston, & Donovan, 1980). Descriptions of temporal rhythm patterns throughout the developmental process and during different crisis experiences have been stated as necessary subsequent research targets. Fitzpatrick has yet to embark upon equally robust research foundations for motion patterns, consciousness patterns, and perceptual patterns.

Fitzpatrick's involvement in graduate nursing education is related to the development of her theoretical views. Her teaching of graduate level nursing theory and nursing research courses has influenced her own and her students' conceptualizations of nursing science and health. Ashworth's (1980), Laffrey's (1982), Loveland-Cherry's (1982), and Reed's (1982) studies are related to health, life perspective, and/or well-being. Doctoral students' attending Fitzpatrick's research-based seminars on rhythmic phenomena have used topics related to rhythmic phenomena for dissertations (Floyd, 1982b; Quillin, in progress). Fitzpatrick's interest in suicidology and gerontological nursing have also played a part in students' selections of research topics.

Nursing interventions have been derived from knowledge arising from the investigations on rhythmic patterns (Fitzpatrick, 1982b). For example, specific indications for reality orientation, rocking, reminiscence, music therapy, and rhythm profiles are supported by certain research findings. With respect to temporal dimensions, identified nursing activities are believed to enhance the meaningfulness of life.

Fitzpatrick's overall model is still in a developmental phase and therefore has yet to have an impact on nursing education. In upcoming years, her ideas about human rhythm patterns and health could fit readily into nursing curricula.

CONCLUSION

A perspective is thought to lead to a knowledge system (Ellis, 1982b). Ellis' (1968) characteristics of significant theories is applied to Fitzpatrick's (1983) ideas and allows conclusions to be drawn about the relevance of the model for nursing. Broadness in scope, complexity, testability, usefulness, implicit values, and information generated are all potentially accounted for in this developing model.

Fitzpatrick's homeodynamic dealings in approaching interactions of person and health permit a broad application and interpretation of nursing phenomena. The abstract diagram of relationships proposed from the model illustrates the potential scope for future investigations in nursing. Concrete credibility is given to a label of "highly complex" via Fitzpatrick's descriptions of person, environment, the indices of holistic human functioning, the meaning attached to life, the domain of health, the manner of coming up with meaningful nursing activities, and the essence of nursing. Even though Fitzpatrick and others have tested fragments of the model, some of the basic relationships have not yet been tested. As shown in the interventions emanating in gerontological counselling (Fitzpatrick, 1982b), Fitzpatrick's model has potential usefulness in guiding the nature and direction of clinical practice. Through its intimate linkage with the meaning attached to life, Fitzpatrick highlights the value of health by means of investigations on suicide and temporal dimensions related to the elderly, the terminally ill, and hospitalized individuals. As a doctoral student, Floyd (1982a) was supported by Fitzpatrick's rhythm research interests in the reformulation of rhythm theories to a psychiatric-mental health nursing application. Fitzpatrick's most notable weakness at this time is parsimony in terminology. Her notion of health implicitly overlaps with a connotation of life perspective. Likewise, perceptual patterns might realistically be embodied within patterns of consciousness.

The process of critical review must continue as new postulations and reformulations of the model are developed. Innovative ways by which to logically challenge theoretical ideas need to be ongoing within the discipline of nursing. Choosing to acknowledge and address these challenges is left for the scientists who focus on theory.

REFERENCES

Alford PA: Temporal experience of individuals in a suicidal crisis. Unpublished Master's research project, Wayne State University, Detroit, Michigan, 1981

Ashworth PE: Health status perception in middlescence I and middlescence II. Unpublished Master's research project, Wayne State University, Detroit, Michigan, 1980

Bentov I: Stalking the Wild Pendulum. Bantam Books, New York, 1977

Bouwman DW: Temporal perspective in middlescence I, middlescence II, and late adulthood. Unpublished Master' research project, Wayne State University, Detroit, Michigan, 1979

Brasuell JM: A comparison of psychological changes produced in aged persons as a result of passage of time, empathetic-clarifying counseling and response-outcome dependence counseling. Unpublished Master's research project, Wayne State University, Detroit, Michigan, 1977

Chaffer NR: Temporal experiences of individuals in a suicidal crisis. Unpublished Master's research project, 1979

Donovan MJ, Fitzpatrick JJ, Johnston RL: Temporal experiences related to the developmental process of aging. Paper presented at the American Psychological Association Convention, Montreal, Canada, September, 1980

Donovan MJ, Fitzpatrick JJ, Johnston RL: Aging, time, and health. Paper presented at the American Psychological Association Annual Convention, Los Angeles, California, August, 1981

Downs FS, Fitzpatrick JJ: Preliminary investigation of the reliability and validity of a tool for the assessment of body position and motor activity. Nursing Research, Vol 25, pp 404-408, 1976

Ellis R: Characteristics of significant theories. Nursing Research, Vol 17, pp 271-222, 1968

Ellis R: Personal communication, May 26, 1982a

Ellis R: Conceptual issues in nursing. Nursing Outlook, Vol 30, pp 406-410, 1982b

Engle VF: A study of the relationship between self-assessment of health, function, personal tempo and time perception in elderly women. Unpublished doctoral dissertation, Wayne State University, Detroit, Michigan, 1981

Fitzpatrick JJ: An investigation of the relationship between temporal orientation, temporal extension, and time perception. Unpublished doctoral dissertation, New York University, 1975

Fitzpatrick JJ: A philosophy of dying. Paper presented at the II International Institute on Health Care Ethics and Human Values, College of Mount St. Joseph, Cincinnati, Ohio, July 12, 1976

Fitzpatrick JJ: Time and motion: Behavioral correlates among the aged. Paper presented at Wayne State University College of Nursing Research Reports, Detroit, Michigan, November, 1977

Fitzpatrick JJ: Possible new variables for assessment and intervention. Paper presented at Indiana University School of Nursing, Seminar in Nursing Futurology, Indianapolis, Indiana, June 13, 1979

Fitzpatrick JJ: Patients' perceptions of time: Current research. International Nursing Review, Vol 27, pp 148-153+, 1980

Fitzpatrick JJ: Is nursing the science of health? Center for Health Research NEWS, Wayne State University, Vol 2, No 2, Detroit, Michigan, 1981a

Fitzpatrick JJ: The essence of nursing. Paper presented at the Lambda Chapter, Sigma Theta Tau Induction Ceremony, Detroit, Michigan, April, 1981b

Fitzpatrick JJ: The path of nursing: The path of science? Unpublished paper presented at The Fourth Annual Nursing Research Symposium, Sigma Theta Tau Nursing Reserach Consortium, Detroit, Michigan, May, 1981c

Fitzpatrick JJ: Toward the future... Center for Health Research NEWS, Wayne State University, Vol 2, No 3, Detroit, Michigan, 1981d

Fitzpatrick JJ: Suicide and temporality: Programmatic research. Paper presented at The University of Iowa College of Nursing, Iowa City, Iowa, May 15, 1981e

Fitzpatrick JJ: Answer 2 to research replication: Questions and answers. Western Journal of Nursing Research, Vol 3, pp 96-97, 1981f

Fitzpatrick JJ: The crisis perspective: Relationship to nursing. In Fitzpatrick JJ, Whall AL, Johnston RL, Floyd JA: Nursing Models and Their Psychiatric Mental Health Applications. Robert J. Brady Co., Bowie, Maryland, 1982a

Fitzpatrick JJ: Techniques of gerontological counseling. In Lego S (ed): Lippincott Manual of Psychiatric Nursing. J.B. Lippincott, Philadelphia, Pennsylvania, 1982b, in press

Fitzpatrick JJ: Visions of nursing. Paper presented at the Doctoral Homecoming, Wayne State University, Detroit, Michigan, May 8, 1982c

Fitzpatrick JJ: A life perspective rhythm model. In Fitzpatrick JJ, Whall AL (eds): Conceptual Models of Nursing: Analysis and Applications, Robert J. Brady Co., Bowie, Maryland, 1983

Fitzpatrick JJ, Donovan MJ: Temporal experiences among hospitalized individuals: A pilot study. Paper presented at The First Sigma Theta Tau Nursing Research Symposium, Wayne State University, Detroit, Michigan, May 13, 1978a

Fitzpatrick JJ, Donovan MJ: Temporal experience and motor behavior among the aging. Research in Nursing and Health, Vol 1, pp 60-68, 1978b

Fitzpatrick JJ, Donovan MJ: A follow-up study of the reliability and validity of the motor activity rating scale. Nursing Research, Vol 28, pp 179-181, 1979

Fitzpatrick JJ, Reed PG: Stress in the crisis experience: nursing interventions. Occupational Health Nursing, Vol 28, pp 19-21, 1980

Fitzpatrick JJ, Whall AL (eds): Conceptual Models of Nursing: Analysis and Applications, Robert J. Brady Co., Bowie, Maryland, 1983

Fitzpatrick JJ, Donovan MJ, Johnston RL: Temporal experiences among terminally ill cancer patients: An exploratory study. Paper presented at The Second Annual Nursing Research Symposium, Sigma Theta Tau Nursing Research Consortium, Ann Arbor, Michigan, May 5, 1979

Fitzpatrick JJ, Donovan MJ, Johnston RL: Experience of time during the crisis of cancer. Cancer Nursing, Vol 3, pp 191-194, 1980

Fitzpatrick JJ, Johnston RL, Donovan MJ: Hospitalization as a crisis: Relation to temporal experiences. Paper presented at The 13th Annual Conference of the Western Society for Research in Nursing, Los Angeles, California, April 30-May 2, 1980

Fitzpatrick JJ, Whall AL, Johnston RL, Floyd JA: Nursing Models and Their Psychiatric Mental Health Applications. Robert J. Brady Co., Bowie, Maryland, 1982

Flaherty GG, Fitzpatrick JJ: Relaxation technique to increase comfort level of postoperative patients: a preliminary study. Nursing Research, Vol 27, pp 352-355, 1978

Floyd JA: Rhythm theory: Relationship to nursing conceptual models. In Fitzpatrick JJ, Whall LA, Johnston RL, Floyd JA (eds): Nursing Models and Their Psychiatric Mental Health Applications. Robert J. Brady Co., Bowie, Maryland, 1982a

Floyd JA: Hospitalization, sleep-wake patterns, and circadian type of psychiatric patients. Unpublished doctoral dissertation, Wayne State University, Detroit, Michigan, 1982b

Fromme SG: The relationship between stated color preference and the vital signs of temperature, pulse rate, and respiratory rate. Unpublished Master's research project, 1979

Goldberg WG, Fitzpatrick JJ: Movement therapy with the aged. Nursing Research, Vol 29, pp 339-346, 1980

Grider JA: A descriptive study of time perception among hospitalized psychiatric patients. Unpublished Master's research project, 1977

Hardy ME: Theories: Components, development, evaluation. Nursing Research, Vol 23, pp 100-107, 1974

Hardy ME: Perspectives on nursing theory. Advances in Nursing Science, Vol 1, pp 37-48, 1978

Haus E: Periodicity in response and susceptibility to environmental stimuli. Annals of the New York Academic Sciences, Vol 107, pp 361-373, 1964

Hartline CA: Temporal perspectives among terminally ill individuals. Unpublished Master's research project, 1978

Horowitz B: Comparison of two relaxation techniques in increasing comfort levels of postoperative open heart surgery patients. Unpublished Master's research project, 1982

Jablonski A: Environmental effects of hospitalization on the mental status of elderly individuals. Unpublished Master's research project, 1978

Johnston RL: Temporality as a measure of unidirectionality within the Rogerian conceptual framework of nursing science. Unpublished doctoral dissertation, Wayne State University, 1980

Johnston RL, Fitzpatrick JJ: Relevance of psychiatric mental health nursing theories to nursing models. In Fitzpatrick AL, Whall RL, Johnston RL, Floyd JA (eds): Nursing Models and Their Psychiatric Mental Health Applications. Robert J. Brady Co., Bowie, Maryland, 1982

Johnston RL, Fitzpatrick JJ, Donovan MJ: Developmental stage: Relationship to temporal dimensions. Paper presented at the ANA Council of Nurse Researchers Annual Meeting, Washington, D.C., September, 1981

Jones EK: A comparison of temporal orientation in elderly institutionalized individuals. Unpublished Master's research project, Wayne State University, Detroit, Michigan, 1977

Kotal BA: Subjective speed of time passage among adults. Unpublished Master's research project, Wayne State University, Detroit, Michigan, 1980

Kuhn T: The Structure of Scientific Revolutions (2nd ed). University of Chicago Press, Chicago, Illinois, 1970

Laffrey S: Health behavior choice as related to self-actualization, body weight, and health conception. Unpublished doctoral dissertation, Wayne State University, Detroit, Michigan, 1982

Loveland-Cherry C: Family system patterns of cohesiveness and autonomy: Relation to family members' health behavior. Unpublished doctoral dissertation, Wayne State University, Detroit, Michigan, 1982

Luce GG: Biological rhythms in psychiatry and medicine. National Institute of Mental Health, U.S. Department of Health, Education and Welfare, Washington, D.C., 1970

Ludwig-Bonney GL: The effect of tape-recorded music on the pain experience of burn patients. Unpublished Master's thesis, Wayne State University, Detroit, Michigan, 1981

Mack H: Temporal experiments among psychiatric patients. Unpublished Master's research project, Wayne State University, Detroit, Michigan, 1978

McDonald S: A study of the relationship between visible lightwaves and the experience of pain. Unpublished doctoral dissertation, Wayne State University, Detroit, Michigan, 1981

Moore G: Perceptual complexity, memory, and human duration experience. Unpublished doctoral dissertation, Wayne State University, Detroit, Michigan, 1981

Nalinnes K: Depression and temporal experience. Unpublished Master's research project, Wayne State University, Detroit, Michigan, 1977

Newman MA: Theory Development in Nursing. F.A. Davis Company, Philadelphia, Pennsylvania, 1979

Pacini CM, Fitzpatrick JJ: Sleep patterns of hospitalized and non-hospitalized aged individuals. Journal of Gerontlogical Nursing, Vol 8, No 6, pp 327-332, 1982

Quillin SM: Growth and development of infant and mother and mother-infant synchrony. Unpublished doctoral dissertation, Wayne State University, Detroit, Michigan, in progress

Ramin CJ: Reminiscence therapy: Changes in morale and self-esteem. Unpublished Master's thesis, Wayne State University, Detroit, Michigan, 1982

Reed PG: Religious perspective, death perspective, and well-being among death-involved and non-death-involved individuals. Unpublished doctoral dissertation, Wayne State University, Detroit, Michigan, 1982

Roberts BL, Fitzpatrick JJ: Vestibular stimulation and balance among the elderly: A pilot study. Accepted for publication in Journal of Gerontological Nursing, 1982

Rogers ME: An Introduction to the Theoretical Basis of Nursing. F.A. Davis Company, Philadelphia, Pennsylvania, 1970

Rogers ME: Postulated correlates of unitary human development. Unpublished course materials, New York University Division of Nursing, 1979

Rogers ME: Nursing: A science of unitary man. In Riehl JP, Roy C (eds): Conceptual Models for Nursing Practice (2nd ed), Appleton-Century-Crofts, New York, 1980

Roslaniec A, Fitzpatrick JJ: Changes in mental status in older adults with four days of hospitalization. Research in Nursing and Health, Vol 2, pp 177-187, 1979

Schorr J: Behavior patterns, temporal orientation and death anxiety. Unpublished doctoral dissertation, Wayne State University, Detroit, Michigan, 1982

Sipols-Lenss M: Vestibular stimulation: Effects on gross motor activity and weight of premature infants. Unpublished Master's thesis, Wayne State University, Detroit, Michigan, 1982

Smith JA: The idea of health: A philosophical inquiry. Advances in Nursing Science, Vol 3, No 3, pp 43-50, 1981

Smokvina GJ: Aging and institutionalization as determinants of temporal and motor phenomena: The data collection process and problems. Unpublished Master's research project, Wayne State University, Detroit, Michigan, 1976

Tillich P: The meaning of health. Perspectives in Biology and Medicine, Vol 5, pp 92-100, 1961

19

NURSING MODELS:
SUMMARY AND FUTURE
PROJECTIONS

Joyce J. Fitzpatrick & Ann L. Whall

As evidenced by the preceding chapters, nursing has a strong and firm foundation in both science and philosophy. The past provides current scholars, philosophers, theorists, researchers, and clinicians with rich resources for present scientific endeavors. The future can be planned based upon knowledge of this strong historical foundation. In fact, as professionals with a committment to society, nurses have a responsibility to plan the future. Hopefully, there will continue to be visionaries among us, those who will not only plan the future, but also create new visions of the possible, who will lead us not only toward new conceptualizations, but also spark innovative strategies of nursing interventions. This summary addresses a few of the trends and issues which have influenced nursing in the past and which will continue to influence nursing in the future. The term nursing science as used in this discussion refers not only to the theoretical knowledge of nursing but also to the investigative processes through which that theoretical knowledge is verified.

Nightingale, in her early nursing model, provides a sound basis for the development of nursing science in her clear statement of the major concepts basic to nursing. The four basic nursing concepts of person, environment, nursing, and health are all included in Nightingale's model. Comparatively less attention is paid, however, to one of the concepts, i.e., person, than to the other three. Nightingale's model in other words is explicitly focused on environment, nursing, and health. The concept of person is, however, central to the implied and stated relationships among the other basic concepts, but the centrality of the concept of person is inferred, rather than explicitly stated by Nightingale. In comparison with some of the later nursing models, Nightingale places relatively greater emphasis on the concept of environment. In her discussion of environmental conditions external to the person, one theme is often identified as a focus on health or on health as an overall nursing goal. Thus, Nightingale influenced the development of later nursing models in terms of identifying major concepts with which nursing is concerned, as well as placing a major emphasis upon the concepts of environment, health, and nursing. Nightingale's influence upon nursing science is evident in terms of both the identification of major theoretical concepts as well as identification of ways in which nursing knowledge may be verified.

In an historical view of the later nursing models, one can identify shifts in the emphasis which is placed upon each of the four basic concepts. A noticeable shift for example is from an emphasis on environment and health, found in Nightingale's model, to an emphasis on nursing, and later to an emphasis on person. In contrast to Nightingale, in the development of later nursing models, the concept of environment is often less of a focus, or at least less explicitly stated. At times this shift of emphasis has occurred because the concept of environment has been subsumed under that of person, e.g., in statements of holistic persons in interaction with environment the two concepts are often blended. At other times there is simply less attention paid to environment as a central concern of nursing.

The later shift in emphasis found in the nursing models to the focus upon the concept of nursing or the nurse/person relationship, is clearly evident in the models developed by Peplau, Orlando, Henderson, and Wiedenbach. Within these models is an emphasis on the therapeutic processes between the nurse and the patient. This focus represents a significant developmental phase in nursing science, that is, nurses were concerned not only with defining the significant scientific content of the discipline, but also with delineating their professional role.

The professional role discussions in the general nursing literature often focus on nursing as intervention. The discussions of the nursing process, for example, often focus greatly upon the nature of the nursing interventions. While there continues to be discussion regarding the centrality of nursing process as a basic nursing concept, the focus on the nursing process (assessment, identification, intervention, and evaluation) is more generally understood to be an example of the application of nursing knowledge to the practice arena. In addition, other discussion continues over whether the central concern of nursing should be on the applied dimension of nursing, i.e., on nursing as verb, as intervention, and/or as a practice discipline. This controversy surfaced early in nursing's scientific development as related to questions of nursing as an applied science. There continues to be a strong emphasis upon the search for prescriptive theoretical approaches. In an overall view of the development of the nursing models the relative importance of the nursing process as a basic concept is unclear.

A more recent shift in emphasis is evident in the focus on person as the central phenomenon of interest to nursing. This focus is most dominant in the model of Rogers. This person focus continues to be particularly clear in those models built upon Rogers, i.e. Newman, Parse, and Fitzpatrick. In these later models, however, one also finds a new, clearer emphasis on the concept of health.

Currently there is considerable scholarly discourse regarding the centrality of/or the focus upon the concept of health in nursing science. The question raised is whether nursing is the science of health. Certainly this can be understood as directly related to the emphasis upon reclaiming Nightingale's wisdom, as well as a search for scientific and professional identity. Any current emphasis on health as the central concept of nursing may also be understood as a developmental stage toward integration and synthesis of the other basic concepts.

More recently the concepts considered basic to nursing, i.e. person, environment, health, and nursing, have been identified through retrospective analyses of the nursing models. During the present time there has also been an increased emphasis upon theory development processes, and more generally upon the development of a distinct body of knowledge within the discipline of nursing. This consciousness regarding the nature of theory development has led to a more explicit identification of theoretical components in the more recently developed nursing models. This consciousness has also led nursing scholars to search for additional commonalities between nursing models.

Thus, there appears to be increasing interest in the commonalities found between models rather than upon exclusive attention to differences between models. Such attention to the commonalities and to the theory development processes is clearly advantageous to the further expansion and refinement of nursing science.

The nursing models examined in this text will continue to have a major influence upon nursing science. If nursing science is viewed as a systematically verified body of knowledge, nursing as a discipline has made much progress. Nursing models are currently being used to develop theories and to guide research and professional practice. Further, new models are being built upon earlier ones and attempts continue to be made to both expand and refine the conceptualizations found in all of the models. Throughout the chapters in this book there are clear examples of the relevance of the nursing models to research, education, and practice. Many more examples can be found in the literature. Undoubtedly, there are also a number of current examples that have not as yet appeared in the nursing literature but which are indicative of the relevance of nursing models to research, education, and practice. It is hoped that the discussions found in this text will provide impetus for new scholarly endeavors, as nurses continue to struggle with clarification of the essence of the discipline.

The future developments within nursing will undoubtedly be based upon an expanded range of existing nursing theory. For example, reformulation of existing theories derived from other disciplines utilizing the nursing models will occur, as well as development of theories from the nursing models, as attempts are made to expand the theoretical base of nursing. Nursing practice will continue to provide examples for scholarly pursuits. As new conceptual leaps are made, new and as yet unknown or unimagined, paths will emerge. Nurse scholars will continue in the persistent quest for knowledge. In its scientific advance it is hoped that nursing will progress toward the goal of science identified by Popper, ". . . towards an infinite yet attainable aim: that of ever discovering new, deeper, and more general problems, and of subjecting our ever tentative answers to ever renewed and ever more rigorous tests" (Popper, p 281, 1959).

REFERENCES

Popper K: The Logic of Scientific Discovery. Basic Books, New York, 1959

INDEX

327

COMPARISON CHART OF NURSING MODELS

NURSING MODELS	DEFINITION OF NURSING	DERIVATION OF NURSING ACTIVITY
Nightingale Chapter 2	A profession for women, the goal of which is to discover and use nature's laws governing health in the service of humanity	To put the person in the best condition for nature to restore or preserve health, and to prevent or cure disease and injury
Peplau Chapter 3	A practice discipline designed to facilitate productive energy transformation	A goal-oriented interpersonal process between nurse and patient
Orlando Chapter 4	Interaction with a patient who has a need, involving patient validation with both the need and the help provided, in order to improve the patient's health	Patient's needs determine nursing acts
Wiedenbach Chapter 5	A deliberate blend of thoughts, feelings, and overt actions . . . practiced in relation to an individual who is in need of help	Patient behavior which indicates a need-for-help triggers nursing activity
Henderson Chapter 6	The assistance of the individual, sick or well, in activities contributing to health or recovery that she/he would perform had she/he the strength, will, or knowledge	Deliberative approach to meet the 14 components of nursing care
Levine Chapter 7	Human interaction; incorporates scientific principles in use of the nursing process	Holistic care individualized to each person's need; nurse supports the person's adaptation
Johnson Chapter 8	Professional discipline with both an art and science component which functions as an external regulatory force for the behavioral system	Nursing activity derives from a need created by a state of instability or disequilibrium in the behavioral system
Orem Chapter 9	A human service designed to overcome human limitations in self-care action for health-related reasons	Nursing acts are derived from judgments as to which patients require nursing, i.e., by the patient's need for therapeutic self-care to sustain life and health
Roy Chapter 10	A process of analyses and action related to the care of the ill or potentially-ill person.	Nursing activity derives from the model which prescribes a process of assessment and intervention. Nursing intervention is carried out within the context of the nursing process and involves manipulation of stimuli.
Paterson and Zderad Chapter 11	Goal-directed response aimed toward nurturing the well-being and more-being of a person with perceived needs related to health/illness	The intersubjective transaction between patient and nurse related to the health/illness quality of living
Neuman Chapter 12	Nursing is a unique profession concerned with the total person, i.e., all the variables affecting an individual's response to stressors	The nurse is an actor, an intervener who acts in relation to either reduction of encounter with stressor or in relation to mitigating the effect of stressors
King Chapter 13	A process of human interaction between nurse and client	Nurse and client perceive each other and the situation, communicate information, mutually set goals and take action to attain goals.
Rogers Chapter 14	A learned profession whose focus is compassionate concern for maintaining and promoting health and caring for and rehabilitating sick and disabled	Seeks to promote symphonic interaction between environment and man (all people in all settings)
Newman Chapter 15	Nursing science focuses on facilitating the health of persons.	Nursing practice assists persons to utilize their own resources to attain higher levels of consciousness
Parse Chapter 16	Science and art focusing on man as living unity	Person's qualitative participation with health experiences
Fitzpatrick Chapter 17	Science and profession which has as its central concern the meaning attached to life (health).	Focused on enhancing the developmental process toward health